Dr. Delgado clearly exp chemicals are responsible exploration of all aspects of intimate imbalance is often the result of the foods we consume, particularly the highly-processed foods that make up the bulk of the average American diet, ultimately causing sexual dissatisfaction or dysfunction. This book will teach you how to reverse these effects and how changing your diet and using specific herbs can change your relationships, making you a star in the bedroom.

John Gray, Author, *Men Are from Mars, Women Are from Venus*

The books written by Nick Delgado, ABAAHP, are for those seeking to sustain a long- lasting loving relationship. If you are struggling with acne, diabetes, heart disease, cancer, weight issues, or fatigue that leads to sexual dysfunction, then you will find out how to be healthier than you've been in your entire life!

Dr. Tami Meraglia, M.D. CEO/Chief Medical Officer
US Stemology Best Selling Author, *The Hormone Secret*

Mastering Love, Sex and Intimacy combines decades of research into an impressive, all-encompassing 21st century guide to happy, loving relationships. The natural solutions in this book will infuse your sex life with love, lust, passion and pleasure, opening the door for you to be an amazing lover. The wisdom shared in this book will help you formulate an unbreakable emotional connection to create soul-level intimacy.

John Abdo Author, *Ultimate Sexual Health & Performance*
- the complete guide to Achieving & restoring Sexual Vitality

i

Dr. Nick Delgado is the 21st Century leader in the use of nutraceuticals to enhance physical relations between men and women and help them understand their own bodies and responses. Wonderful experiences result from following his guidelines to developing understanding of a partner's body, as well as emotional and psychological needs. This is the definitive instruction book for the care and expanding of your love life.

He explores all aspects of intimate relationships – he clearly explains how hormones and chemicals often control physiological responses. This book also delves into the science of nutrition and how the types of foods we put into our bodies can improve or sometimes destroy our bodies' abilities to achieve lasting and frequent sexual satisfaction. From the biochemistry of love and addressing sexual dysfunction, to how to be an amazing lover and create a deep, emotional bond – this is a definitive guide to happy and enjoyable sexual passion.

Mastering Love, Sex & Intimacy

The New Guide to Pleasure for Men and Women

Nick Delgado, Ph.D., ABAAHP

A power of mind hypnosis script for sizzling sex

(Adult Only) link at the end of this text to Online Course

Mastering Love, Sex & Intimacy
The New Guide to Pleasure for Men and Women
By Nick Delgado, Ph.D. ABAAHP

© 2019 Nick Delgado
Published by Health Wellness Studios Inc.
160 Greentree Dr. # 101 Dover, DE 19904

ISBN: 978-0-9962196-1-7

This publication contains the opinions and ideas of its authors. It is intended to provide helpful and informative material on the subjects addressed in the publication. It is sold with the understanding that the authors and publisher are not engaged in rendering medical, health, or any other kind of personal professional services in the book. The reader should consult his or her medical, health, or other competent professional before adopting any of the suggestions in this book or drawing inferences from it.

The authors and publisher specifically disclaim all responsibility for any liability, loss, or risk, personal or otherwise, which is incurred as a consequence, directly or indirectly, of the use and application of any of the contents in this book.

Foreword

I really wanted to fix our relationship, but our marriage was failing. I was trying desperately to do everything right as a husband, but I was going about it in all the wrong ways. I wanted to be an amazing lover and rock my wife's world but like too many men, I really had no clue how to properly satisfy a woman.

I'll never forget the pain and shame that I felt the day she told me I was a lousy lover. My inability to please my wife made me feel inadequate -- like I had completely failed as a man. I felt like hiding under a rock in shame and was terrified that she was going to leave me for a better lover. I didn't want to be heartbroken and alone and was desperate for a solution.

Then, as if by chance, something amazing happened...

In learning about the role of sex hormones and biochemistry at a conference, my interest was piqued, and I became obsessed with finding safe and effective ways to boost testosterone and growth hormones. My research also led to discovering the vital roles that estrogen and nitric oxide play in sexual functioning, and over a dozen other chemicals that influence love, lust, sexual health, and pleasure.

It became crystal clear to me how to use performance enhancing chemistry to enhance heighten or enrich intimacy and become an amazing lover. I decided to use this knowledge to not only save my own relationship but also help other men who were struggling with the same issues or who wanted to learn how to become super heroes in the bedroom.

I read every book on relationships, love, and sex that I could get my hands on. I discovered that how you engage a woman's mind is just as important as how you interface with her body; that you need to not only perform better but connect with her emotions as well. I also learned how to deepen the love connection with sensual massages, Kundalini, non-sexual touch, open communication, the languages of love, and a variety of other techniques that lead to a lasting, loving relationship.

I applied what I learned in my own relationship to my wife's great pleasure and I also began counseling other couples and. I was shocked to learn how many of the women I was counselling were not having consistent orgasms and how many of them admitted to "faking it." In researching this issue, I realized there is a lack of knowledge and importance placed on the female orgasm, and that saddened me. I became an expert in female anatomy and learned all about physical, chemical, psychological, and emotional inhibitors of female pleasure. And I discovered key principles that both men and women can use, allowing for full surrender and ecstasy and multiple orgasms in women.

As I applied and practiced this knowledge, I no longer felt like less than a man; I felt like a legendary lover. I incorporated all of this knowledge into my counselling sessions and achieved consistently amazing results. Both the men and women experienced a dramatic improvement in their sex lives, and a deeper level of intimacy. And their relationship satisfaction scores skyrocketed.

But there was still a problem. . .

There were no real supplements on the market with the type of clinical benefits required to match the case studies. So I spent years developing my own, which not only matched the potency of many pharmaceuticals but exceeded them. The nutraceuticals that I developed are far safer, have fewer side effects, and (unlike most pharmaceuticals) they can be taken on an ongoing basis without losing efficacy over time.

I wanted to share what I had learned on a global scale and help both men and women overcome lackluster sex lives, sexual dysfunction, biochemical imbalances, and emotional barriers to love. I wanted everyone to experiences the depths of ecstasy that only knowledge and true intimacy can provide. So I started writing my own book and filled it with the secrets I had been proving were correct for over four decades.

But I didn't stop there. I realized it was going to take more than a book - there needed to be a human element as well. I thought if I could create something that would make it possible to heal relationships through amazing sex leading to better love and intimacy, I'd be really happy. My team and I worked hard to combine everything we had learned and proven (in our own lives, in the lab and in clinical practice) into an online course. The *Love, Sex and Intimacy* course shares all the secrets to mastering biochemistry and creating a deeply satisfying relationship and sex life.

Because there are often emotional and psychological factors that inhibit pleasure and intimacy and can prevent people from applying our teachings, we also developed a form of hypnosis that bypasses these shortcomings, even for the most difficult of cases.

After 40 years of research and development, 20 years of field testing, five years of focused organization, and two years of programming, we finally put this all together. During that time, I have helped more than 2000 couples transform their relationships. all of the information you need to transform your own sex life and relationship is here. My team and I are excited to finally present this definitive twenty-first century guide to Mastering Love, Sex, and Intimacy.

Contents

Introduction

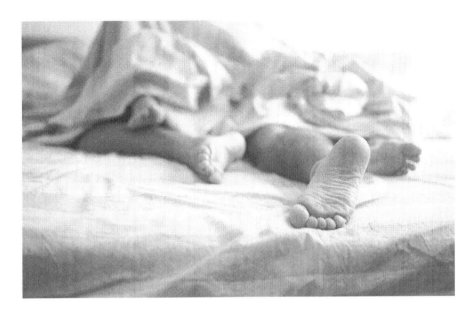

Amazing, connected, and orgasmic sex is the most blissful experience both men and women can have in life, and it is the glue that holds happy couples together. Sex is ideally enjoyed daily, yet a mere 4% of Americans report actually doing so.[1] Once a month is kind of the average for those over the age of 45, and personally I think that that's a disconnect from the human need for touch, sex, and love. When I ask my clients in long-term relationships about their sex life, many say to me "I still love my partner, but we just don't have sex that often." And my response is always - "Why?"

Seeing just how uncommon mutually satisfying, daily sex is in America saddens me. A whopping 41% of men and 27%

---

[1] https://today.yougov.com/news/2017/08/29/most-americans-want-have-more-sex/?belboon=031b3908984b04d39400589a,4711850,subid=100097X155 5749X6b48ed68e0f8813c97edf7a6c5de32de&pdl.rlid=203577

of women report being sexually dissatisfied, and a mere 30% of women report having an orgasm every time.[23] Women are also faking it a whole lot -- 67% of them admit to faking it either occasionally or always![4] And the stats are equally dismal for the elderly -- only 57% of adults over 60 report being sexually active.[5] Clearly there is something amiss here.

Physical health, biochemistry, mental and emotional blocks, sexual attitudes, and cultural assumptions, all play a role in the creation of these statistics. I wrote this book because I believe that a euphorically satisfying sex life and deep level of intimacy should be enjoyed by all adults, and they are achievable regardless of age, gender or health status. The following information is derived from decades of research on sexual health and pleasure. I have condensed all of this information into an easy-to-follow guide, so that you and your partner can have the mind-blowing sex lives and emotional and spiritual intimacy that you both deserve!

[2] https://www.ncbi.nlm.nih.gov/pubmed/26900897
[3] http://abcnews.go.com/images/Politics/959a1AmericanSexSurvey.pdf
[4] http://www.apa.org/monitor/2011/04/orgasm.aspx
[5] https://www.ncbi.nlm.nih.gov/pmc/articles/PMC3267340/

The Many Benefits of Sex

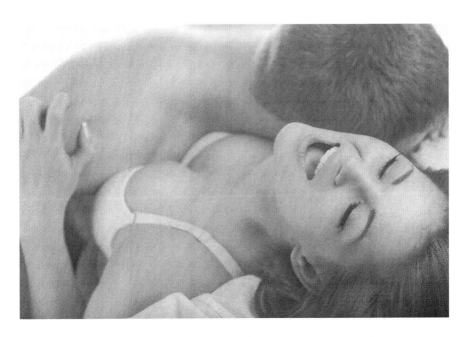

It's easy for couples to fall into a rut, and sexual frequency often declines after the initial honeymoon phase wears off. Frequency also tends to decline with age, but these two things are choices, not something that you are doomed to. Having more sex increases the *desire* to have more sex (this is a scientifically proven fact by the way), so if you're continually "not in the mood," I recommend you do it anyway. Your partner will appreciate it, and you may just find that you are the one initiating sex the next time around.

Aside from conception, pleasure is the main motivation behind sex, and this book will help you to maximize it. But sex is not merely about pleasure -- it is also important for your health and essential for the health of your relationship. Below is a list of the top, scientifically proven benefits of sex. I suggest you refer to these benefits if you experience any resistance to implementing the guidelines in this book. Some of the guidelines may not be easy to follow at first, but the payoff will be well worth it.

Relationship Benefits

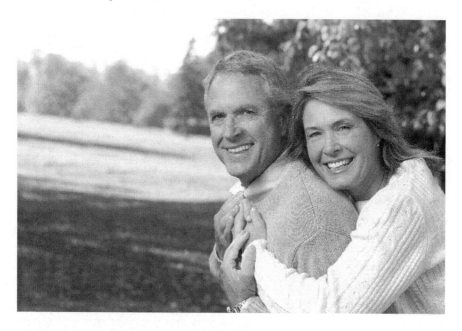

Couples who report greater sexual frequency and satisfaction have a much higher chance of remaining in a long, stable, and happy relationship, and there is a notably lower divorce rate among them. There is also a dose-dependent relationship -- the more sex a couple has, the happier they claim to be together. Sex helps you feel more connected and closer to your partner and strengthens the bond between you. The intimacy of the act itself helps you reconnect, and it separates couples from mere roommates.

According to large-scale studies, couples who have a healthy sex life are also more satisfied and content with their relationship. One reason for this is that reaching orgasm causes a release of the love hormone oxytocin -- which is a key formulator of love, trust, bonding, and connectivity. Oxytocin also helps promote positive relationship behaviors such as listening, laughing, and affirming. The enhanced communication that it promotes reduces tension and stress between couples, leads to fewer arguments, and makes conflict resolution a whole lot easier.

Mental and Emotional Benefits

Having sex helps to release endorphins that flush the stress hormone cortisol from the body, which markedly reduces stress and anxiety levels. Being physically and emotionally close with another human being also helps enhance feelings of security and wellbeing, which leads to increased happiness levels and a reduced risk for depression. The mere sight of your lover triggers the release of PEA hormone, which is a hormone that makes people feel attached and happy. Sex also helps remind you of your masculinity/femininity and sexuality, makes you feel desirable, and in the context of a relationship, makes you feel loved and accepted -- all of which enhance self-esteem.

Physical Benefits

Sexual arousal and intercourse both help to naturally increase testosterone levels, a deficiency common in aging men and women. Testosterone enhances sexual function and libido and helps to increase bone and muscle mass, promote fat loss, brighten mood, and increase memory as well. Sex also releases beta-endorphins and other natural painkilling chemicals in the brain that help to reduce both chronic and acute pain. It has been found to be particularly helpful for relieving pain associated with headaches, migraines, and arthritis.

Orgasms increase DHEA which helps boost immunity and cognitive capabilities, promote healthy, youthful looking skin, increase and balance sex hormones, fight sexual dysfunction, repair damaged tissue, and fight depression. Orgasms also cause the release of prolactin, melatonin, and oxytocin -- all of which promote relaxation, and a deep, restful sleep. The effects of prolactin seem to be stronger in men than in women, which could be because many women don't orgasm during sex, and/or because the levels of prolactin released in men may be higher.

Sex also helps enhance heart health by lowering blood pressure and stress, which are two major risk factors for heart disease. In fact, according to a 10-year-long study conducted at Queen's University in Belfast, having orgasms at least twice a week cuts the risk of heart attacks and stroke in half. Preliminary research suggests sex may also help enhance prostate health. One study found men who ejaculate at least 21 times a month (from sex or masturbation) have a significantly lower risk of prostate cancer than men who ejaculate four to seven times per month.

Sex is also an enjoyable form of exercise – it helps increase heart rate and burns approximately five calories a minute. It makes you smarter too! Research shows regular sex increases brain activity and may even bolster brain growth, critical thinking capabilities, concentration, and intelligence levels. If all that weren't enough, sex can help prevent you from getting sick. According to research conducted at Wilkes University in Pennsylvania, people who have sex two or more times weekly have 30% higher levels of the immune-boosting, infection-fighting antibody-immunoglobulin A.

Anti-aging Benefits

"I say that physical intimacy and exercise are your best defense against aging and bad health. This potent duo is a far cheaper prescription than any skin-enhancing cosmetic cream you can buy or any pill in your bathroom." -- *Secrets of the Superyoung by David Weeks*

Sex helps to slow the inward and outward signs of aging by boosting anti-aging hormones. After an orgasm, the wrinkles on your face are reduced, and you are left with a youthful afterglow. Sex that is physically active also releases a small amount of HGH, which is an anti-aging hormone that enhances skin elasticity. And the effects are notable: according to a study published in the book *Secrets of the Superyoung*, improving the quality of one's sex life can help a person look between four and seven years younger.

Longevity Benefits

Regular sex helps to reduce the risk for nearly every deadly chronic disease, and studies have proven beyond a doubt that regular sexual intimacy increases longevity. Inhabitants of the longest living populations in the world tend to fall in love early and maintain an interest in sex throughout their lives. And there appears to be a dose-dependent relationship between sex and longevity -- the more sex a person has, the lower their risk of death.

Sex dramatically reduces stress levels which is beneficial because stress damages DNA, lowers the immune system, increases your risk for chronic disease, and can shave between four and eight years off your life expectancy. Sex also helps to stimulate and balance neurotransmitters and hormones that affect longevity.

Part 1
The Underlying Causes of Sexual Dysfunction and a Lackluster Love Life

Chapter 1
The Most Common Types of Sexual Dysfunction

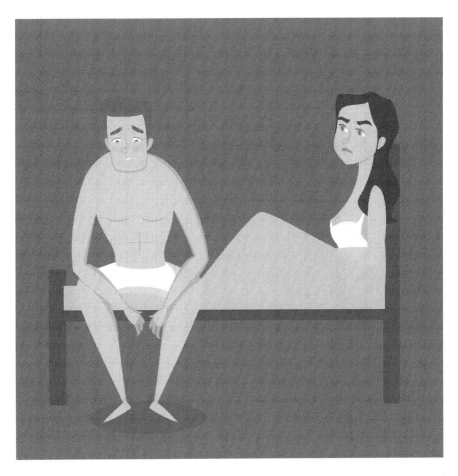

Sexual dysfunction is any mental, emotional, or physical problem that prevents you or your partner from receiving sexual satisfaction. It is quite common in both men and women, and most will experience it at some point in their lives.

The Most Common Types of Sexual Dysfunction in Women Include:

Low Sexual Desire

This is the most common type of female sexual dysfunction and approximately 43% of women worldwide experience it.[6]

Lack of Lubrication

The second most common sexual dysfunction in women. Lack of lubrication can occur at any age, but it is most common in menopausal and postmenopausal women. It affects 56% of women over the age of 40.[7]

Arousal Disorder

An inability to become aroused during sexual activity affects approximately 17% of females.[8]

Orgasmic Disorder

This dysfunction is characterized by recurrent difficulty in achieving orgasm, in spite of sufficient sexual arousal and ongoing stimulation. Approximately 10%

---

[6] http://www.soc.ucsb.edu/sexinfo/article/low-sexual-desire

[7] http://www.healthywomen.org/content/article/menopause-and-your-sexual-health-when-dryness-equals-discomfort

[8]

http://www.nejm.org/doi/full/10.1056/NEJMcp050154?viewType=Print&viewClass=Print&

of women have orgasmic disorder, and 5% never achieve orgasm at all.[9]

Sexual Pain Disorder

Worth noting: what is perceived as female "sexual dysfunction" may have absolutely nothing to do with the female's psychology or physiology. A lack of desire, arousal, lubrication, and an inability to orgasm may simply be the result of a selfish or unknowledgeable lover or the vaginal orgasm myth (which I'll get to later).

The Most Common Types of Sexual Dysfunction in Men Include:

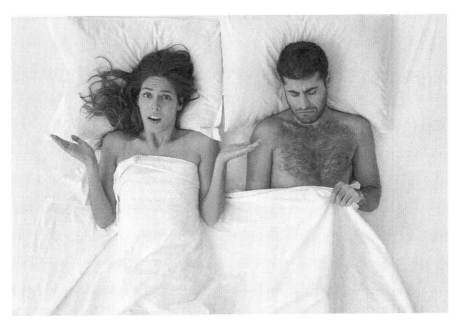

---

[9] https://www.psychologytoday.com/blog/all-about-sex/200903/the-most-important-sexual-statistic

Erectile Dysfunction

Erectile dysfunction, or ED, is the inability of a man to achieve or to maintain an erection. It is the most prevalent form of sexual dysfunction in men, and it is astonishingly common. Approximately 26% of men under 40 report experiencing either partial or complete ED, and that number rises to 40% by the age of 40 and to 70% by the age of 70. [10] [11] The underlying cause of ongoing adult ED is often physiologically based; however, it can be caused by psychological factors as well. Fortunately, the condition is almost always treatable, and the holistic lifestyle medicine approach outlined in this book is far more effective at reversing it than prescription medications such as Viagra® (which is effective a mere 30% of the time).

Loss of Desire

A lack of sexual desire is most often associated with women, but men experience it just as frequently as women in heterosexual relationships.[12] According to a National Health study of American men, 15% of men between the ages of 18 and 59 have "persistent

---

[10]

http://www.clevelandclinicmeded.com/medicalpubs/diseasemanagement/endocrinology/erectile-dysfunction/

[11] http://onlinelibrary.wiley.com/doi/10.1111/jsm.12179/abstract

[12] Davies, S., Katz, J., & Jackson, J. L. (1999). Sexual desire discrepancies: Effects on sexual and relationship satisfaction in heterosexual dating couples. Archives of Sexual Behavior, 28, 553-567. doi: 10.1023/A:1018721417683

complaints of low sexual desire."[13] The majority of men in this study blamed medical (medications, depression etc.) and biological reasons for their low libido, but psychological reasons, such as stress or attitudes towards sex can also be to blame.

Ejaculatory Disorders

The most common ejaculatory disorder is premature ejaculation, which every man has experienced at one time or another (see Chapter 11 for treatment methods). Other types of ejaculatory disorders include delayed ejaculation, anejaculation (a complete inability to ejaculate), perceived ejaculate volume reduction (ejaculating less semen than previously), and decreased force of ejaculation. Both biological and psychological factors can trigger the first three types of ejaculatory disorders, while biological factors alone are usually the cause of the last two.

---

[13] Rosen, R. (2000) Prevalence and risk factors of sexual dysfunction in men and women. Current Psychiatry Reports, 2, 189-195. doi: 10.1007/s11920-996-0006-2

Chapter 2
Psychological Causes of Sexual Dysfunction and An Unsatisfying Sex-life

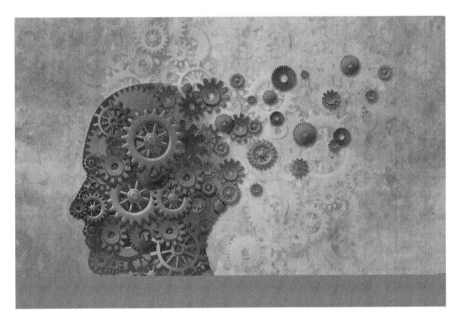

In order to restore libido and prevent or reverse any type of sexual dysfunction, you need to first identify the underlying cause, and often there is more than one factor at play. While most holistic-oriented practitioners appreciate the power of biochemistry, hormones, supplements, diet, and exercise for healthy sexual functioning, many fail to address the power of the mind. This is unfortunate because sex starts in the brain, and psychological issues are a common cause of sexual dysfunction and sexual dissatisfaction.

Top Psychological Causes:

Self-Esteem and Body-Image Issues

Poor self-esteem is a major sexual sabotager. It can prevent you from communicating your sexual needs, preferences, fantasies and desires with your partner. It can also prevent you from initiating sex, experimenting in the bedroom, and from letting go and getting out of your head during the act. If you have body image issues, worrying about your appearance and/or trying to hide your body stops you from being in the moment, and this negative thinking can make the whole experiencing undesirable.

All of the above factors reduce your ability to experience pleasure and can diminish your desire to engage in sex. They can also lead to vaginal dryness and pain in women, ED and ejaculatory problems in men, and inhibited orgasms in both genders.

Poor self-esteem can also prevent you from attracting a sexual partner in the first place. A recent survey asked 17,000 women what trait they found sexiest, and 65% said confidence, while only 7% said wealth![14] Although I couldn't find a large-scale study to prove how desirable self-confidence is to men, I'm sure the correlation is equally strong. Men love ladies who have that "Je ne sais quoi," that intangible self-assurance that comes through in the way they walk, talk, and act that makes them extremely desirable and irresistible.

Loving yourself and your body requires both physical and mental work. You need to respect and take care of your body to truly love and embrace it. Consuming a healthy diet and

---

[14] https://priceonomics.com/the-united-states-of-sex-a-survey-of-17000-women/

exercising regularly will help you to achieve a healthy body, which will make you more confident in life and in between the sheets. If you are unsure of what exactly a healthy diet entails because of all the conflicting information out there, or you want to learn how to make meals that are both nutritious and delicious, you can purchase a copy of the *Simply Healthy Cookbook* on our site.

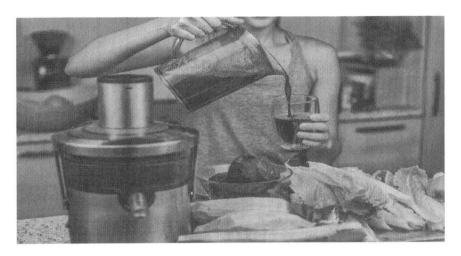

While it is important to actively work towards your ideal body weight for sexual and health purposes, you should not put off embracing your body and feeling sexy or having great sex until you reach it. You have a choice to feel bad or ashamed of your body or to love and accept it, right now in this moment. Start by shutting down self-criticisms and letting go of the need for outside approval. Don't listen to any negative messages from others or from the media.

Get comfortable with your body by spending as much time naked as possible. Practice gratitude for all that your body does for you – and spend time daily focusing on what you love about your body. While having sex, focus on the pleasure sensations that your body is providing you and your partner.

Another tip from sex expert Susan Bratton is to use an orange light in place of your regular light bulb – it acts as a beautifier and illuminates the body in the most gorgeous way possible.

Pay attention to your inner dialogue and replace negative words and thinking with positive ones – this is necessary for both enhancing confidence and eliminating body image issues. Positive affirmations, hypnosis, guided meditations and LFC Audio Scripts can help you with this. You can also improve your self-esteem by being more assertive, trying new things, doing activities you enjoy, facing your fears, avoiding comparing yourself to others, writing down and working towards goals, and practicing forgiveness (of self and others).

Stress and Adrenal Fatigue

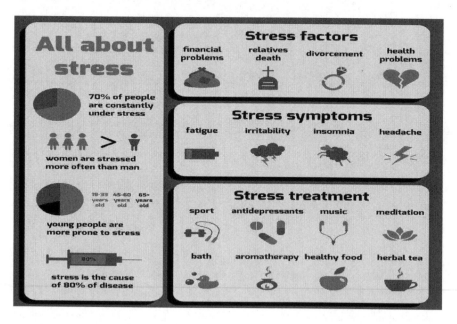

Approximately 70%-80% of Americans report feeling stressed frequently throughout their day, and this stress transfers into the bedroom. Stress hinders sexual functioning by causing fatigue, throwing sex hormones out of whack, making you moody and irritable, and reducing oxytocin (which is the bonding, love hormone). A few examples of common sources of stress include work, traffic, long lines, the Western diet (especially sugar and stimulants), bills, interpersonal upheavals, worries about your children's safety, and marital problems.

The adrenal glands help you cope with stress, and if you experience chronic high stress levels or have experienced a major trauma, it is likely that your adrenal glands, which are responsible for producing stress and sex hormones, are fatigued. The adrenal glands play a crucial role in sexual function and libido.

When your adrenal glands are fatigued, your body goes into survival mode and shuts down non-essential functions, which includes the production of sex hormones. You lose your passion for life, your passion for your partner, and your sex drive becomes negligible.

To reverse the sex-sabotaging effects of stress and adrenal fatigue, you need to address both outside stressors and inner, emotional stressors.

While you may not be able to completely avoid stressful situations, you can control how you perceive and react to them and dramatically reduce the amount of stress they cause your body. Becoming more positive and optimistic and consciously focusing on all the good things in life is tremendously helpful. Try keeping a gratitude journal and writing down five or ten things you are grateful for every day. Daily meditation, Emotional Freedom Technique (EFT), breathwork therapy, EMDR therapy, self-hypnosis, and my personal favorite, LFC eyes-open hypnosis scripts (available at

Delgadoprotocol.com) are also excellent tools for reducing stress, clearing out past traumas, and cultivating positivity.

Also, look for blessings in the little things, in all the moments throughout your day. Notice and appreciate the smile on your lover's or child's face, appreciate how your dog greets you, how nice your sheets feel, the hot water running over your body in a shower, and even the physical ability to move. If you find you are always in a time-crunch, teach yourself time-management skills. Most of us have more free time than we realize, but we waste it on things such as social media or TV.

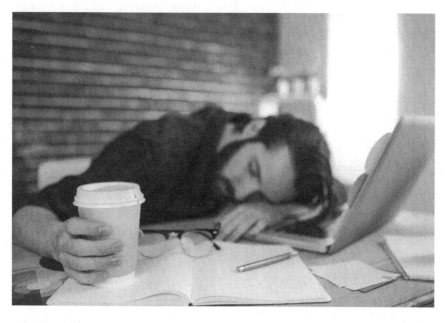

Another way to reduce stress is to spend five minutes at the end of each work day jotting down anything that is bothering you, making 'to-do' lists for the upcoming day, and noting five things that you are grateful for. Delegation at home and at the workplace can also help. Learning to say no is absolutely essential. High quality sleep is also essential for managing stress and restoring adrenal health. Watching sunsets is beneficial because it resets your circadian rhythm helping you fall asleep more easily. Practice sleep hygiene by sleeping in a cool, dark, and silent environment, and keeping all electronics out of the bedroom.

You should also eliminate alcohol, refined carbs, artificial sweeteners, vegetable oils, processed foods, foods you are intolerant to, and stimulants such as caffeine and sugar which cause physical stress and tax the adrenal glands. And try to eat something every three hours, consume complex carbohydrates combined with either healthy protein or fat at each meal, and avoid caffeine, refined carbohydrates, sugar and other stimulants. Eating this way will help to balance your blood sugar and reduce the stress load on your adrenal glands.

If you are suffering with low energy and other adrenal fatigue symptoms (anxiety, loss of sex drive, lightheadedness, brain fog, difficulty getting up in the morning, poor immunity, salt cravings etc.), I recommend you also take Adrenal DMG. Adrenal DMG contains a blend of adrenal cortex, apoptogenic herbs, and other clinically proven nutrients for supporting adrenal function and boosting cortisol production. Many of my clients report enhanced well-being and energy, as well as an increased ability to cope with stress almost immediately after starting it (see appendix for more on Adrenal DMG).

Relationship Drama

When there is a lot of stress or drama in a relationship, it often stems from a failure of one or both of the partners to listen to and absorb what the other is saying. We are frequently so caught up in "winning" the argument that, instead of listening, we are merely waiting for our next opportunity to talk. Next time you and your partner are in the middle of a discussion or argument, pay attention to what your partner is saying, and instead of interpreting the words through your own biases, try to interpret them as a third party would. If you find it difficult to admit when you are wrong, or you are tempted to interrupt your partner, or to rehash old arguments, repeat the following question in your mind "Would I rather be right, or be happy?"

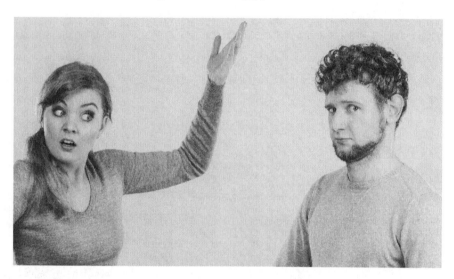

Remember no one is perfect; accept your partner's flaws and focus instead on all the wonderful things that made you fall in love with him or her. Often times what bothers you most about other people are things you don't like about yourself. See your partner as a reflection of yourself, and if there is something about your partner that agitates or triggers you, resist the urge to project and look inwards instead.

Another major source of stress is misunderstanding or misinterpreting your partner's words or actions. *The 5*

Languages of Love is a book and website filled with tons of useful and free information on enhancing communication and better understanding of your partner.[15] Other leading sources of relationship stress that may need to be addressed include emotional baggage from childhood or past relationships, failure to fully commit, holding onto grudges or failing to forgive, an imbalance of chores that should be shared, lack of trust, failing to take care of oneself, codependency, lack of boundaries, criticism, neglecting to prioritize valuable time together, and last but not least, a lack of frequent, mutually satisfying sex.

Depression

Depression is extremely common, and it can have a cyclic effect on your relationship: the depression causes an emotional and physical disconnect from your partner, and the disconnect worsens depression. Depression is a major inhibitor of libido which can be caused by mental and/or physical imbalances and also by unaddressed emotional traumas. Unfortunately, allopathic doctors treat all depressed patients under the assumption that they have a neurotransmitter imbalance (which is often not the case), and the medications they prescribe can significantly decrease libido, arousal, and orgasm frequency and intensity.[16]

If you experience ongoing depression, it is advised that you see a naturopath or functional medicine practitioner to reverse chemically-based depression. The practitioners of these professions take a holistic approach and aim to address the underlying cause with safe and natural methods. And if a

---

[15] http://www.5lovelanguages.com/
[16] https://www.ncbi.nlm.nih.gov/pmc/articles/PMC3108697/

neurotransmitter imbalance does happen to be at play, they will treat it with herbs and other nutraceuticals that are natural and free of sexual side-effects.

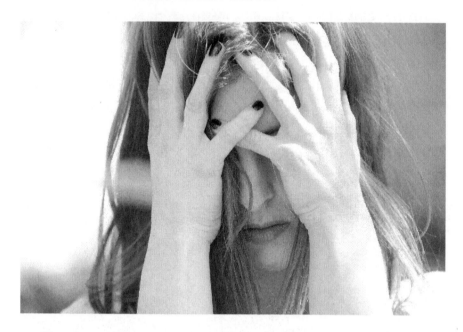

If the depression is rooted in past trauma, a hypnotherapist, therapeutic breathwork facilitator, or NLP practitioner can help to reverse the mentally and emotionally-rooted depression. Worth noting is that low testosterone can lead to depression, and if you experience it in conjunction with sexual symptoms, you should have your total testosterone levels measured. If they are low or on the low-end-of-normal, Testro Vida Pro or Testrogenisis cream can help optimize your testosterone levels and maximize your libido and virility (see appendix).

Past Sexual Trauma

Sexual trauma during youth is frighteningly common in both genders -- one in four girls and one in six boys will experience it before the age of 18.[17] It is also very common in college-aged women, with 23% experiencing some form of sexual assault.[18] Unfortunately, recovery isn't easy, and most survivors don't take the necessary steps to achieve it. If left unaddressed, sexual trauma can cause a total loss of desire, or reduced sensations of pleasure, painful sex, an inability to orgasm, and/or erectile dysfunction. It can also lead to sexual promiscuity, recklessness, sexual addiction, emotional numbness and unfulfilling, disconnected sex.

Sexual trauma frequently interferes with the ability to trust and may even cause you to feel anger towards your partner for desiring or initiating sex.[19] It can also cause you to associate feelings of shame with sex and pleasure. And the loss of personal power and control that occurs can cause you to over-assert yourself in every aspect of your relationship and prevent the surrendering that is necessary for sexual pleasure and release.[20]

To recover from sexual trauma, you need to realize you are not alone, you did not cause the assault, and there is no shame in what happened to you. Also, you cannot recover on your own, and suffering in silence will harm your mental, emotional and physical wellbeing. It is important that you open up and share your experience with a family member or close friend, and that you talk to your lover about it. You may also require professional help. A qualified and experienced

---

[17]

https://www.nsvrc.org/sites/default/files/publications_nsvrc_factsheet_media-packet_statistics-about-sexual-violence_0.pdf

[18] https://www.rainn.org/statistics/campus-sexual-violence

[19] https://www.psychologytoday.com/blog/all-about-sex/201609/childhood-sexual-abuse-sexual-recovery-is-possible

[20] https://www.psychologytoday.com/blog/all-about-sex/201609/childhood-sexual-abuse-sexual-recovery-is-possible

clinical hypnotherapist or NLP practitioner can be especially helpful because they can quickly access the subconscious mind where memories and traumas are stored.[21] [22] Tantric sex can also be tremendously helpful, and we will explore it further in Chapter 15.

Additional Psychological Causes

The above are the leading psychological causes of sexual dysfunction, but there are numerous others that can be at play. Additional common contributors include performance anxiety, sexual guilt and shame (learned from parents or through religious or societal training), an overly- analytical mind, pornography addiction, marital problems, and a lack of understanding of you or your partner's body. It's important to note that there is often more than one psychological issue that needs to be dealt with, or there is a combination of physical or biochemical and psychological culprits that need to be addressed.

---

[21] https://www.ncbi.nlm.nih.gov/pubmed/2664731
[22] http://personis.co/healing-from-trauma-and-abuse-with-nlp/

Chapter 3
Physical Causes of Sexual Dissatisfaction and Dysfunction

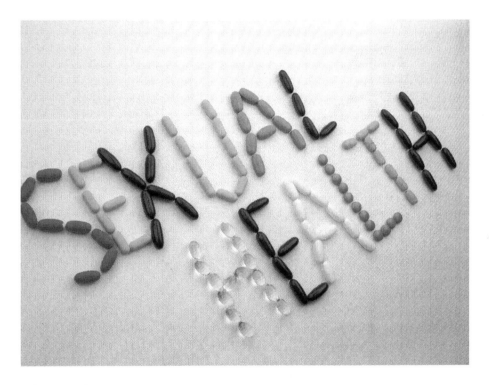

Clogged Arteries

Clogged arteries occur when fats and cholesterol (primarily from vegetable oils and animal products such as eggs, dairy, poultry and meat) build up in your artery walls. High-fat foods elevate triglycerides, thicken the blood, increase blood pressure and diabetes risk, and accelerate the thickening of the arteries to the heart and sex organs.

In order to experience pleasure and reach orgasm, blood and oxygen must first flow to your sex organs. When your arteries are clogged, the passageway for blood flow is narrowed, and the reduced flow caused by even mildly clogged arteries reduces the ability to experience arousal, pleasure, and orgasm in both genders. It also reduces a male's ability to perform sexually and is a leading cause of ED and ejaculatory disorders in men. If the buildup of plaque progresses too far, it can lead to a complete inability to achieve an erection.

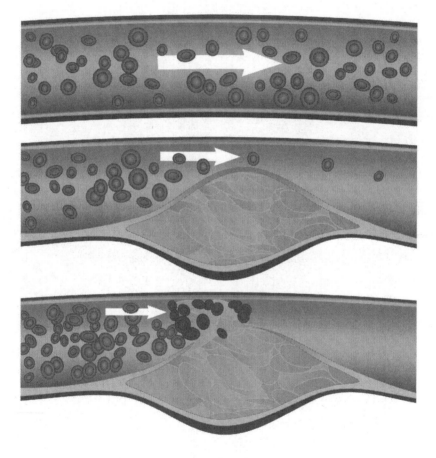

Every year past the age of 35 increases the probability of accumulating plaque in the arteries to the sex organs, heart, and brain. Unfortunately, most people don't realize they have clogged arteries, and failure to identify and treat the condition dramatically increases heart attack and stroke risk. If you have high blood pressure, high cholesterol and high triglycerides (after fasting or after eating), plus sexual symptoms with no other identifiable cause, then it's highly likely that you have clogged arteries. And if you are male with the aforementioned symptoms plus ED, then it's almost guaranteed that your arteries are substantially clogged. The penile arteries are a mere two mm in diameter, while the coronary artery is seven to eight mm in diameter; therefore, it takes a lot less arterial plaque to notice penile symptoms of clogged arteries than it does for heart symptoms to appear. In this instance, ED is actually a blessing in disguise because it serves as an early warning sign of vascular disease.

The best way to clean-up your arteries is to combine a plaque-clearing diet with a special supplement called <u>PCOS Heart Plus</u> (see appendix for more information). For tons of useful free tips on the ultimate libido boosting, plaque-clearing diet (which is centered around plant proteins and the removal of all processed oils), see my <u>Youtube Channel</u> titled "Dr. Nick Delgado." You'll also find information on this channel on how to get your protein, fiber, and essential fatty acids requirements met with delicious, satisfying plant foods.

Too Much PDE-5 (Men)

cGMP is an enzyme that helps to relax the smooth muscles and is required for blood to flow to the penis and for an erection to occur. PDE-5 is an enzyme that often increases with age, and it degrades, or breaks down cGMP. Too much PDE-5 is therefore a major cause of sexual dysfunction, and prescription medications such as Viagra® work by reducing the ability of PDE-5 to degrade cGMP.

The reason why Viagra® and other PDE-5 inhibiting drugs are only effective in approximately 30% of patients is because nitric oxide, or NO, is required for the production of cGMP. Aging and lifestyle factors can lead to a depletion of NO, and ironically enough, PDE-5 inhibiting drugs such as Viagra® use up the supply of NO with each use, which can lead to an NO deficiency. This also explains why PDE-5 inhibitors may work initially, and then spontaneously stop working: because their continued use depletes NO stores. Without enough NO, all the cGMP in the world will not yield an erection.

Herbs and nutrients that may help reduce PDE-5 include horny goat weed (epimedium), Tongkat Ali, pomegranate, and cinnamon.[23] According to *Longevity Medicine Review*, 2018, the amino acids l-arginine and l-citrulline may also help to boost NO, and to not only manage, but reverse erectile dysfunction in men with heart disease, type-2 diabetes or plaque buildup.[24] The scientific review states these amino acids can provide systemic sexual performance benefits, and they do so safely and without producing any negative side-effect.[25]

What may be more effective than even the "Blue Pill"?

Try **Amore** for men and **Passion Pill** for woman. Amore and Passion Pill are not available online, only by request to

---

[23] https://www.ncbi.nlm.nih.gov/pmc/articles/PMC2483323/

[24] http://www.lmreview.com/articles/print/l-citrulline-restoring-erectile-function-viagra-doesnt/

[25] http://www.lmreview.com/articles/print/l-citrulline-restoring-erectile-function-viagra-doesnt/

email Admin@delgadoprotocol.com or calling 1-949-720-1554 PST 9:30 a.m. to 4:30 p.m.

When you use the Blue Pill or Amore, it is best to add Beet Vitality for the best amino acid and Nitric oxide restoration: https://delgadoprotocol.com/product/beet-vitality/

*see appendix for more information on these two products

Poor Liver Health

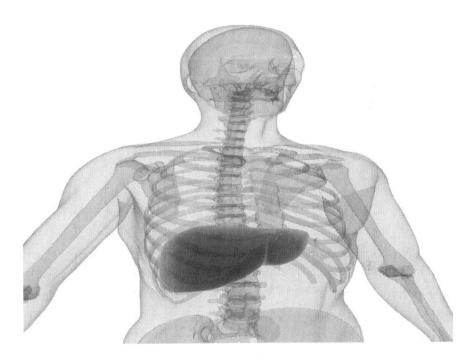

The liver plays a key role in metabolizing and detoxifying toxins and excess estrogens. Over time the liver function can become compromised and its ability to metabolize estrogens reduced. The build-up of toxic estrogens can then trigger or worsen estrogen dominance (see Chapter 6) and its sexual symptoms. Liver disease is associated with a loss of libido, testicular shrinking, breast enlargement, and a significant reduction of both total and free testosterone levels.[26] [27]And the effects aren't subtle: one study found over 50% of men with liver cirrhosis experience feminization and erectile dysfunction.[28]

Poor liver health can also affect sexual functioning on an energetic level. In Taoism and Traditional Chinese Medicine (TCM), it has long been taught that the liver controls the flow of sexual energy or chi, in the body. According to TCM a weakened liver can result in a reduced flow of energy to the genitals and difficulty with achieving orgasms.[29] [30]

To enhance your liver health, consume a whole-foods, plant-based diet, eliminate or reduce alcohol and sugar, and take Liv D-Tox (see appendix for more information).

Brain Injury

The pituitary gland is a pea-sized gland located at the base of the brain. It is often referred to as the "master gland" because it produces critical hormones and also controls the hormone-generating glands in your body, including the thyroid, adrenals, testicles and ovaries. Traumatic brain injury (TBI) can damage the pituitary gland and cause several hormone imbalances, and according to one study, 30% of TBI patients experience pituitary damage.[31]

The sex hormone imbalances that pituitary damage often leads to can cause several sexual symptoms including

---

[26] https://www.nature.com/articles/3901316
[27] https://www.ncbi.nlm.nih.gov/pubmed/1874492
[28] https://www.nature.com/articles/3901316
[29] https://agelessherbs.com/liver-qi-stagnation/
[30] https://www.yinovacenter.com/blog/reviving-your-sex-drive/
[31] http://mnfunctionalneurology.com/hormones-whack-since-brain-injury/

impotence, reduced fertility, and altered sex drive.[32] The injury itself may be big or small; and some common causes include sports-related injuries, falls, car accidents, domestic violence, or simply an accidental blow to the head. Sometimes the symptoms won't show up until weeks or years later, and the incident may not even be remembered making it difficult to make the connection. Worth noting, with mild brain injury the damage may not be identifiable with conventional medical screening tools, but the patient may suffer with hormone imbalances and sexual difficulties nonetheless.[33] [34]

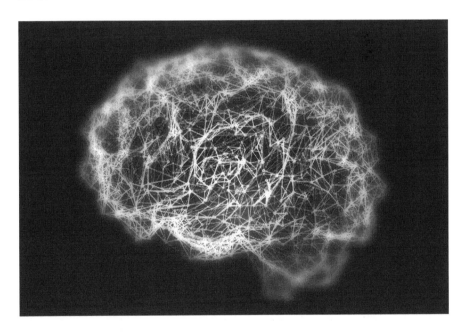

If you have experienced any type of head injury, work with a functional medicine practitioner to identify and correct

[32] https://www.hormone.org/diseases-and-conditions/pituitary/traumatic-brain-injury

[33] https://www.hormone.org/diseases-and-conditions/pituitary/traumatic-brain-injury

[34] https://www.headway.org.uk/about-brain-injury/individuals/effects-of-brain-injury/hormonal-imbalances/

potential hormone imbalances. If hormone replacement therapy is needed, use bioidentical hormones because they are safer, have fewer side-effects, and are typically more effective than synthetic hormones.

Prescription Medications

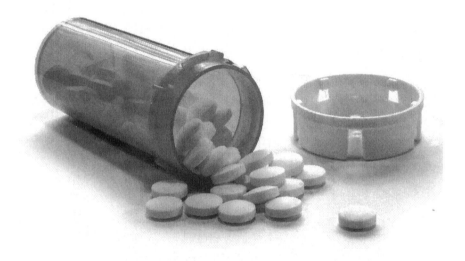

Approximately 70% of Americans are currently on at least one prescription drug, many of which cause sexual side-effects.[35] Some of the most commonly prescribed medications that can cause sexual dysfunction include antidepressants, antipsychotics, statins and fibrates, blood pressure medications, opioid pain medications, anti-seizure medications, benzodiazepines (tranquilizers and anti-anxiety drugs), birth control pills, anticonvulsants, and

---

[35] https://www.sciencedaily.com/releases/2013/06/130619132352.htm

antihistamines.[36] It is important that you never stop a prescription medication on your own and that you work alongside a qualified practitioner when doing so.

Mattresses and Other Xenoestrogens

Mattresses? What can they have to do with sexual dysfunction? In 2007, it became mandated that all US mattresses must contain enough fire-retardant chemicals to withstand a two-foot wide blowtorch open flame for 70 seconds. These chemicals are not only sprayed on mattresses, they are also commonly used on couches, car seats, building insulation, and electronics. Fire retardant chemicals are highly toxic, and our continuous exposure to them causes a toxic build-up in the body. These endocrine disruptors burden the liver and contribute to estrogen dominance (more on this in Chapter 6) and other hormone irregularities – all of which can lower libido and lead to sexual dysfunction.[37] Brominated fire retardants can also trigger sexual dysfunction in a less direct way by damaging the thyroid gland, adrenal glands, and cardiovascular health.[38] [39] If money permits, find a mattress that meets the US flammability standard with non-toxic materials such as wool.

Additional Possible Causes

Other factors which may lead to sexual dysfunction include chronic diseases (such as obesity, diabetes, and

---

[36] https://www.aarp.org/health/drugs-supplements/info-04-2012/medications-that-can-cause-sexual-dysfunction.html

[37] https://www.nature.com › scientific reports › articles

[38] https://www.sciencedaily.com/releases/2016/04/160404091227.htm

[39] www.issm.info/sexual...qa/can-thyroid-problems-contribute-to-erectile-dysfunction-ed/

atherosclerosis), incompatible pheromones, smoking, alcohol abuse, poor oral health (15% of men with ED suffer from periodontitis), pelvic floor weakness (kegels are beneficial for both genders), job dissatisfaction, insomnia and other sleep disorders, and a lack of clitoral stimulation in women (most women can't orgasm from intercourse alone).

Chapter 4
Chemical Causes of Sexual Dissatisfaction and Dysfunction

Hormone Imbalances

HORMONES

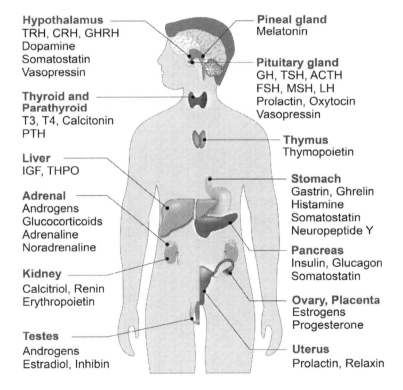

Hypothalamus
TRH, CRH, GHRH
Dopamine
Somatostatin
Vasopressin

Thyroid and Parathyroid
T3, T4, Calcitonin
PTH

Liver
IGF, THPO

Adrenal
Androgens
Glucocorticoids
Adrenaline
Noradrenaline

Kidney
Calcitriol, Renin
Erythropoietin

Testes
Androgens
Estradiol, Inhibin

Pineal gland
Melatonin

Pituitary gland
GH, TSH, ACTH
FSH, MSH, LH
Prolactin, Oxytocin
Vasopressin

Thymus
Thymopoietin

Stomach
Gastrin, Ghrelin
Histamine
Somatostatin
Neuropeptide Y

Pancreas
Insulin, Glucagon
Somatostatin

Ovary, Placenta
Estrogens
Progesterone

Uterus
Prolactin, Relaxin

The following hormones play a leading role in sexual functioning, libido, arousal, attachment and bonding:

Biochemistry refers to the chemical processes that occur within the body, and biochemical imbalances are a very common cause of sexual dysfunction. Several hormones and neurotransmitters are required for libido and sexual functioning, and an imbalance of any one of them can have a major negative impact on your sex life and your personal life. In this chapter we will explore the most common biochemical causes of sexual dysfunction, and in Chapter 5, I will teach you how to reverse the imbalances.

Testosterone

Although it is often thought of as a male hormone, testosterone plays a major role in sexual health for both men and women. Testosterone levels progressively decline after the age of 20 and deficiencies are extremely common. Testosterone can give you the drive and confidence to pursue your partner in the early stages of love, and it helps keeps the passion alive in long-term love. If you experience a low libido or sudden loss of sexual desire, or if you are a male who experiences erectile dysfunction, you should consider having your total testosterone levels checked (see Chapter 6 for information on how to boost testosterone).[40]

Oxytocin

Oxytocin is the love, connectivity, and bonding hormone (it also acts as a neurotransmitter), and it is released during intercourse and orgasms. Oxytocin helps to increase sexual desire and intensity, it aids in the release of dopamine, and

---

[40]

https://www.betterhealth.vic.gov.au/health/conditionsandtreatments/androgen-deficiency-in-women plays a key role in multiple orgasms in women.[41] It also causes muscle contractions and sensitizes nerves and preliminary research suggests increasing oxytocin may help produce more intense orgasms.[42] Oxytocin is required to feel empathy, intimacy, and a connection and bond with your partner; it heals and holds a relationship together, and a deficiency can make sex feel mechanical and impersonal.

Oxytocin has natural antidepressant properties and is often referred to as the "cuddle hormone" because it is released through touch. It is responsible for the wonderful, relaxed feeling and sense of wellbeing you experience after a massage, a long hug, or a snuggle session with your significant other. Women naturally release much higher levels of oxytocin, which is why many women find it difficult to not get emotionally involved with someone they are sexually intimate with.

DHT

Dihydrotestosterone, or DHT, is an extremely potent sex hormone that an enzyme called 5α-reductase synthesizes from testosterone. DHT helps create strong erections and powerful orgasms, and it plays a key role in ejaculation in men. Its sexual effects in women are less pronounced, but it plays a role in the development of pubic hair and breast growth during puberty.[43] You need to maintain DHT within a delicate range, because if it rises too high, acne, hair loss (male and female pattern baldness), prostate enlargement can develop.

---

[41] "The Neurobiology of Sexual Function." Cindy M. Meston, PhD, Penny F. Frohlich, MA

[42] https://www.livescience.com/44574-oxytocin-sex-orgasm.html

[43] http://www.yourhormones.info/hormones/dihydrotestosterone/

DHEA

Produced by the adrenal glands, DHEA also plays a key role in sexual desire, arousal, and function. One of the reasons DHEA is so important for a sexually healthy relationship is because it is a precursor to all of the sex hormones, including testosterone.[44] DHEA also converts into androstenedione, which is an extremely potent pheromone found naturally in sweat.[45] Pheromones are powerful catalysts of sexual chemistry and play a key role in who you are attracted to, and who you attract.

Vasopressin

Vasopressin is another hormone that plays a vital role in attachment, bonding, commitment, and monogamy, especially in men. Elevating vasopressin can turn even the most promiscuous alpha male into a possessive, one-woman-man. It takes approximately 30 consecutive days of sexual intimacy for vasopressin to kick in for a man, and once it does, the urge to bond with the woman who releases it becomes irresistible.

Vasopressin causes a man to let his guard down, quashes the urge to wander and be with other females, and makes him crave the women he is with.[46] It also causes him to unconsciously view his woman territorially and to associate her with "home."[47] Not surprisingly, studies show if a man or woman has fewer receptor sites for vasopressin and oxytocin, it can interfere with their ability and desire to form a monogamous relationship.

---

[44] http://clinchem.aaccjnls.org/content/46/3/414
[45] http://clinchem.aaccjnls.org/content/46/3/414
[46] http://www.eoht.info/page/Neurochemistry
[47] https://www.ncbi.nlm.nih.gov/pmc/articles/PMC3537144/

Vitamin D Deficiency

Most people don't realize this, but vitamin D functions as a hormone in your body. Ever notice that you tend to feel friskier in the summer or during a sunny vacation? This is no coincidence. Vitamin D3 plays an essential role in libido and sexual functioning. It increases Luteinizing Hormone (LH) levels, and LH helps you release testosterone. Low D3 can also lead to an estrogen deficiency in women, and too little estrogen is just as much of a libido killer as too much. Restoring vitamin D levels may also help reduce cortisol output. This is beneficial because elevated cortisol is a major libido killer, and cortisol is produced at the expense of testosterone, so chronically high levels can contribute to a testosterone deficiency.

Growth Hormones (Men)

Growth hormones naturally decline with age, and their decline is blamed for many aging-related symptoms. Studies suggest that growth hormones play a role in the sexual response of the male genitalia and are required for erectile function.[48] Growth hormones also help to optimize the production of nitric oxide and to enhance the volume and firmness of the erections.[49] According to hormone specialist Dr. Thierry Hertoghe, increasing growth hormones also leads to prolonged erections and enhances the effectiveness of other types of hormone therapy.[50]

Thyroid Hormones

---

[48] https://www.ncbi.nlm.nih.gov/pubmed/23014134
[49] https://clinicaltrials.gov/ct2/show/NCT00470002
[50] https://www.youtube.com/watch?v=gNeaPuzxXfl

THYROID DISEASE — ICONS SET

Symptoms of HYPOthyroidism

WEIGHT GAIN

INFERTILITY

IRREGULAR MENSTRUAL PERIODS

HYPERTENSION

ELEVATED CHOLESTEROL LEVEL

CONSTIPATION

DRY SKIN

PAIN OR SWELLING IN JOINTS

IMPAIRED MEMORY

THINNING AND HAIR LOSS

INCREASED SENSITIVITY TO COLD

SLOWED HEART RATE

symptoms of HYPERthyroidism

TACHYCARDIA

AN ENLARGED THYROID GLAND (GOITER)

INCREASED APPETITE

DIFFICULTY SLEEPING

FREQUENT BOWEL MOVEMENT

VISION CHANGES

DIZZINESS

SUDDEN WEIGHT LOSS

Thyroid diseases are associated with sexual dysfunction, and symptoms such as a diminished ability to become aroused, less pleasurable sensations to the genitals, loss of libido, infertility in both genders; miscarriages and vaginal dryness in women; and reduced ability to achieve or maintain erections, delayed ejaculation, and/or decreased sperm count in men.[51] Hyperthyroidism (an overactive thyroid) and hypothyroidism (an underactive thyroid) are two common types of thyroid disease and if left untreated both can also lead to testosterone and estrogen deficiencies, which results in additional sexual side-effects.

Additional Hormones

Other hormones that can lead to sexual dysfunction that you may want to be tested and treated for include cortisol (too high or too low), estrogen (see Chapter 6), SHBG (too much causes a deficiency of testosterone), and prolactin (too high or too low).[52]

Visit https://delgadoprotocol.com/ **to take our free hormone quizzes and find out what you and your partner can benefit from.**

Neurotransmitter Imbalances

Neurotransmitters are chemical messengers that communicate information throughout your brain and body. When hormone therapy fails to treat sexual dysfunction, it is usually because the brain (which is the most important organ

---

[51] https://www.pennmedicine.org/updates/blogs/womens-health/2016/july/how-thyroid-problems-might-be-hurting-your-sex-life

[52] https://www.ncbi.nlm.nih.gov/pubmed/24345293

for a healthy sexy life) has been neglected. A variety of neurotransmitters influence desire, arousal, and orgasms. We will explore the leading neurotransmitters below, and in Chapter 5, I will share tips on how to optimize these neurotransmitters.

Nitric Oxide

Nitric oxide, or NO, is a molecule that sends signals throughout your entire body, helping your 50 trillion cells communicate with each other. Nitric oxide levels typically begin to decline in your mid- to late 20s and continue to decline by approximately 10% to 12% per decade. NO is the ultimate pleasure molecule, and it plays several key roles in sexual functioning, desire, and arousal.

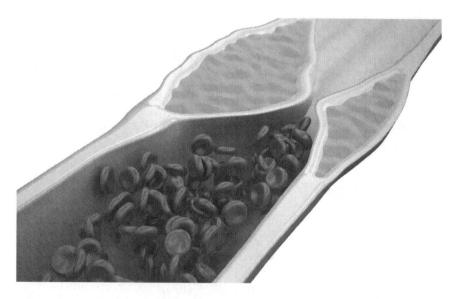

In order for arousal to occur, blood must first flow to the sexual organs. Low nitric oxide levels cause the blood vessels to restrict, encourage red blood cells to clump together, and create dangerous blockages and clots in the arteries. These factors combined dramatically reduce the flow of blood to the sex organs, lowering sensations of pleasure, and interfering with the ability to become aroused and reach orgasm in both genders.

Without enough NO, blood flow to the clitoris is inhibited. Increasing NO cannot only enhance sensitivity, but also increase lubrication and make orgasms more intense and easier to achieve for women. Low NO is also a chief cause of erectile dysfunction (ED) in men because NO is required for blood to fill the erectile body. Optimized NO levels in men allows the muscles in the penis to fully relax and blood to engorge the chambers, leading to enhanced firmness, sensation, and pleasure. And the more blood that fills and stays in the chambers, the larger and firmer the penis becomes.

In many cases, boosting NO is all that is required for restoring pleasure and arousal in both men and women and reversing ED in men. Increasing NO also reduces the risk for, and slows the progression of, cardiovascular disease, hyperlipidemia, diabetes, hypertension, atherosclerosis, and Alzheimer's disease, to name a few.

*Refer to our appendix for information on our nitric oxide boosting supplements

Dopamine

Dopamine plays a key role in pleasure, motivation, and addiction. Dopamine levels rise during sexual arousal, and they flood the brain at the time of orgasm. Dopamine enhances your receptivity to pleasure, and without enough you may experience a low libido, no motivation to pursue or partake in sex, lethargy, an inability to feel love or attachment, and lackluster or absent orgasms. Dopamine also plays a complex but important role in the production of testosterone, which is considered the most important hormone for sexual desire and pleasure. While low dopamine is a more common cause of sexual dysfunction, too much dopamine can also be problematic and may cause premature ejaculation, sexual addiction, aggression, and psychosis.

Serotonin

Serotonin plays a key role in regulating mood and emotions, and too much or too little can impact your sex life. A healthy level of serotonin helps to reduce anxiety, promote relaxation and optimize desire and responsiveness. When serotonin levels are too high, it diminishes sexual desire and arousal, reduces clitoral pleasure, inhibits or reduces the intensity of orgasms, and can lead to ejaculatory disorders.[53] This is why SSRI medications, which increase serotonin and are frequently prescribed for depression, often produce sexual side effects. Excessive serotonin can also blunt emotions, which interferes with romantic love and can prevent feelings of attachment.[54]

If serotonin levels drop too low, the physical drive for sex will likely increase; however, mental and emotional disruptions which interfere with seeking and receiving pleasure may occur. Low serotonin is associated with anxiety, depression, irritability, aggression, low self-esteem and negative thinking.[55]

---

[53] https://www.medscape.org/viewarticle/482059
[54] https://www.medscape.org/viewarticle/482059
[55] https://www.ncbi.nlm.nih.gov/pmc/articles/PMC2077351/

PEA

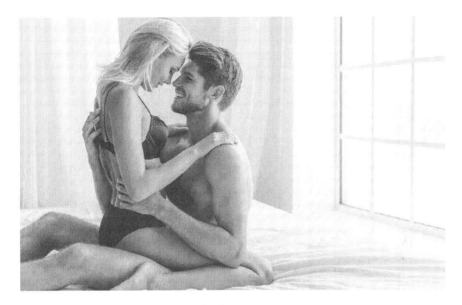

PEA (phenylethylamine) is the best-known, naturally occurring lust chemical, and it is released in largest amounts when you first fall in love. It promotes feelings of infatuation, focused attention, giddiness, uncertainty, euphoria and insatiable desire for your new partner. PEA also intensifies the action of the four important love chemicals: dopamine, serotonin, norepinephrine (a stimulant that enhances alertness and the ability to recall even the most minute details about your significant other), and acetylcholine (a neurotransmitter that plays a key role in arousal, passion, focus, and memory, and is required for erections).

Additional Neurotransmitters

Additional neurotransmitters that can lead to sexual dysfunction or dissatisfaction include epinephrine (too low), and histamine (required for arousal).[56] Neuro Insight™ is a unique supplement that helps to balance and optimize a range of important neurotransmitters by contributing methyl donors, which are substances that donate methyl groups required for the production of neurotransmitters. Please refer to the appendix for more information on this nutraceutical.

---

[56] https://www.ncbi.nlm.nih.gov/pubmed/7770195

Part 2
Natural Solutions for Optimizing Sexual Health, Libido and Performance

Chapter 5
Optimizing Love Chemicals for Greater Intimacy, Connectedness, and Passion

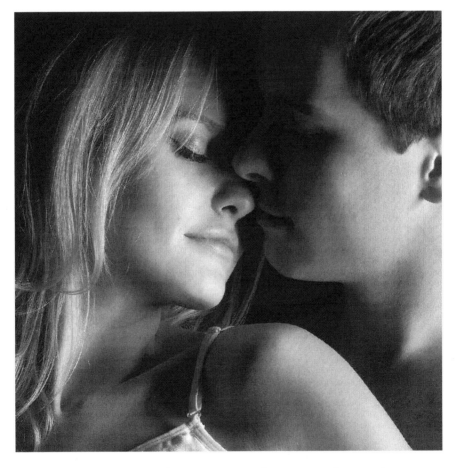

The love, intimacy, connectedness, and passion new couples typically experience are some of the greatest feelings available to mankind. Sadly, as relationships progress, one or all of these feelings often deteriorates, and the result is either relationship dissatisfaction or termination. The good news is that these feelings are fueled by chemicals in your body and stimulating these natural love chemicals can restore the sizzle in your relationship. In Chapter 4 I shared with you the most common biochemical causes of sexual dysfunction, and in this chapter, I will show you how to optimize those chemicals.

Hormones

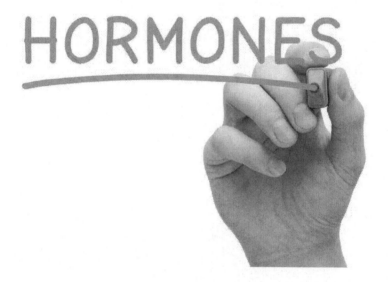

Oxytocin

Sexual frequency often declines as a relationship progresses, and many couples lose touch with the need for physical affection, touching, and intimacy. A reduction of orgasms and lack of touch dramatically reduces oxytocin levels and can make you feel disconnected from your partner. The disconnectedness often leads to a further decline in sexual activity and touch, which creates a negative cycle that can sabotage a relationship and/or cause a person to seek love from an outside source. Fortunately, the solution is simple -- all you have to do is make hand-holding, hugging, kissing, and cuddling a priority, and commit to having more sex.

Even if you don't feel like it initially, having sex will increase the desire to have more sex, so just go for it! Increasing direct eye contact (especially during sex), meditating, non-sexual touch with friends, and sensual massages are also excellent ways to boost oxytocin.

*We work with doctors who can prescribe oxytocin. 50 Units dissolved under the tongue, 30 minutes prior to sex, can help a woman to more easily reach orgasm and a man to be more loving, relaxed, receptive and connected. For more information send us an email at: admin@delgadoprotocol.com

DHT

Women generally don't need to worry about low DHT levels, and men need to keep their DHT within a delicate range. If tests indicate a deficiency of DHT, you can boost it by lifting heavy weights, reducing body fat, and increasing testosterone with an herbal supplement that also contains zinc, such as Testro Vida Pro (see appendix).

If levels are too high in men or women (a common sign of high DHT is balding around the temples), then consume an alkalizing, high-vegetable diet with plenty of lycopene-rich foods (tomatoes, watermelon, carrots and mangoes). The supplement DHT Block can also help bring DHT into a healthy range, and promote a balancing of other hormones that are important for sexual functioning.

DHEA

A decline in DHEA is one of the reasons why sex often becomes less of a priority in aging adults and restoring youthful levels can dramatically enhance a flailing sex life. Because DHEA is produced in the adrenal glands, supporting adrenal health with stress reduction, high quality sleep, and the elimination of refined carbs and sugar can help to increase DHEA. Healthy fats such as coconuts, avocados, olives, nuts and seeds are also beneficial.

An herbal adrenal boosting supplement that contains adaptogens and adrenal cortex can also help increase DHEA and is especially useful if you experience ongoing fatigue. For a more pronounced and immediate effect, you can use Testrogenesis Cream which contains DHEA and a blend of other essential nutrients for sexual health.

Vasopressin

Vasopressin is one of the less well-known love chemicals, and aside from having sex for an extended length of time, there has not been much research on how to increase it or stimulate its release. However, preliminary evidence suggests saunas, the consumption of salt (be careful with this one since most Americans already consume too much), and exercise may help raise vasopressin levels.[57] Supplements that contain Rhodiola, Ginkgo, and/or Berberine, may also help increase vasopressin according to preliminary research.[58] [59] [60]

---

[57] https://www.ncbi.nlm.nih.gov/pubmed/1834624
[58] https://www.ncbi.nlm.nih.gov/pubmed/17295371
[59] https://www.ncbi.nlm.nih.gov/pubmed/10077434
[60] https://www.ncbi.nlm.nih.gov/pubmed/15643562

Vitamin D

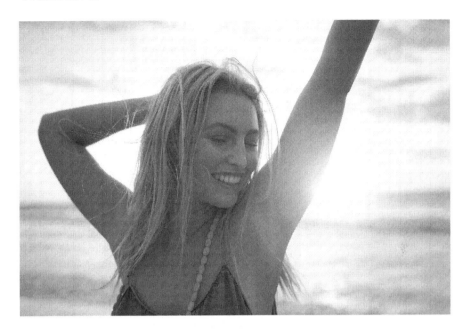

To increase vitamin D, try to get 15 minutes of sunlight exposure on unprotected skin daily. If that is not possible, consider using a sunlamp for 20-40 minutes a day, or taking D3 supplements that provide 2,000 IU per serving.[61] The vast majority of Americans are deficient in vitamin D, but it is possible to overdose on vitamin D supplements, so have your levels tested before supplementing. Vitamin D-rich foods are also beneficial; some good sources include mushrooms, mackerel, sardines, halibut, salmon, trout, and tuna. Don't overdo it with seafood though (no more than 1 to 2 servings a week) because most seafood is contaminated with mercury and other heavy metals.

---

[61] https://www.drweil.com/vitamins-supplements-herbs/vitamins/vitamin-d/

Growth Hormones

To enhance growth hormones, reduce sugar intake, partake in high intensity exercise, lose excess body fat, get more sleep, and take Grow Young spray. Grow Young is a sublingual growth factor spray, and it contains protein peptides that safely stimulate your body's own release of growth hormones.

Thyroid Hormones

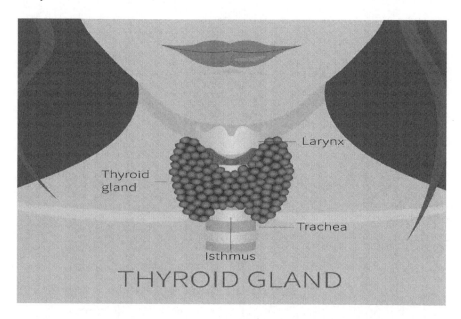

Larynx

Thyroid gland

Trachea

Isthmus

THYROID GLAND

If you suspect you may be suffering with thyroid hormone imbalances, have a full thyroid panel done (most doctors will only test TSH, which fails to identify many thyroid disorders). The panel should test TSH, Free T4, Free T3, Reverse T3, Thyroid Peroxidase Antibodies, and Thyroglobulin antibodies. You should also have your iodine levels checked because an iodine deficiency is a major cause of hypothyroidism (underactive thyroid). A combination of lifestyle modifications and nutraceuticals can reverse most cases of hyperthyroidism (overactive thyroid) and hypothyroidism, and if you suffer with either, I recommend you have a functional medicine practitioner create a customized recovery program for you.

Neurotransmitters

Nitric Oxide

To boost nitric oxide (NO), follow the diet and lifestyle guidelines provided later in this book, and be sure to consume beets, leafy greens, dark chocolate, pomegranate juice, watermelon, citrus, lettuce, garlic and walnuts. Optimizing sleep, exercising regularly, regular sunlight exposure, and reducing blood pressure and cholesterol levels will also help boost NO. If you really want to turbocharge your sex life, I recommend you also take an NO-boosting supplement such as Beet Vitality or Stay Young (see appendix). Many of my patients report noticing increased desire, arousal, and sexual performance on the very first day of starting these products!

Dopamine

If you have low dopamine, it is best to boost it using natural methods – this will optimize dopamine without causing it to become too high. Some ways to increase dopamine include reducing stress, trying new things, exercising regularly, partaking in rewarding activities and/or things that make you feel a sense of achievement, and listening to music. Also eliminate saturated fats, sugar and artificial sweeteners, and consume tyrosine-rich foods. Tyrosine is an essential building block of dopamine, and some healthy sources include bananas, nuts, seeds, beans, legumes, spirulina, and soy. Natural supplements can also be helpful, and you may want to talk to your healthcare practitioner about taking l-tyrosine, Rhodiola, or Mucuna pruriens.[62] [63] [64]

Serotonin

Some natural techniques for boosting low serotonin levels include exposure to bright light (either with the sun or a sun lamp), aerobic exercise, enhancing gut health with probiotics, and addressing negative subconscious thinking patterns that impact your mood with self-hypnosis or LFC glasses.[65] You can also boost serotonin by consuming a diet that is rich in whole food-based complex carbohydrates such as chickpeas, legumes, beans, potatoes, and squash; and tryptophan-rich foods such as soy, walnuts, leafy greens and sea vegetables.

The most common cause of high serotonin levels is SSRI medications in combination with various other prescription drugs. If your levels are elevated, the easiest solution is to discontinue the medication that is causing the excessive serotonin levels and use natural methods to boost serotonin instead. This should never be done abruptly, or on your own however; it should only be done under the supervision of a Naturopathic Doctor or other qualified healthcare practitioner.

PEA

Unfortunately, PEA wears off after a period of time with a new partner, which can range from three weeks to three years,

---

[62] https://www.ncbi.nlm.nih.gov/pubmed/15643562
[63] https://www.ncbi.nlm.nih.gov/pubmed/10077434
[64] https://www.ncbi.nlm.nih.gov/pubmed/17295371
[65] https://www.ncbi.nlm.nih.gov/pmc/articles/PMC2077351/strogen

and lust and passion often fade with it. PEA can be addictive for some, causing them to bounce from relationship to relationship in search of a PEA high. And the common adage "I love him/her, but I am no longer in love with him/her" is usually a result of a PEA decline.

The most important thing you can do here is to recognize that PEA levels will inevitably decline in any relationship, and it is not a reflection of your partner, compatibility, chemistry or relationship quality. It is also essential that you formulate an emotional bond during the initial stages of a romance, because that bond is what will keep you together once the PEA-induced butterflies and euphoria fade. You can also get a mild PEA boosting effect by consuming phenylalanine rich foods such as cocoa, cacao nibs, beans, lentils, nuts and seeds.

Chapter 6
Balancing Testosterone and Estrogen Levels For Better Sex and Fertility

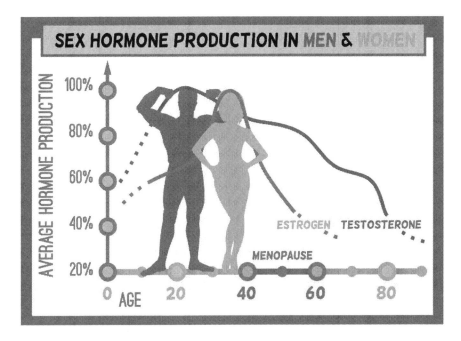

SEX HORMONE PRODUCTION IN MEN & WOMEN

Too much or too little estrogen and/or too little testosterone can inhibit sexual desire, function, and fertility in both genders. Because they play such an integral role in sexuality, I've dedicated an entire chapter to them.

How to Reverse Estrogen Dominance

Because of the modern diet and lifestyle as well as overexposure to xenoestrogens (environmental estrogen-like compounds), many people struggle with excessive estrogen in their systems. This condition is called estrogen dominance. It can also develop when progesterone drops too low, even if estrogen levels are in the normal range, because progesterone keeps estrogen in check. Estrogen dominance is rarely diagnosed and is especially common in people who are overweight, and in women in their 30s and early 40s. It is also quite common in aging men -- most men past 50 have more estrogen than do 25-year-old women! Estrogen dominance can cause mood swings, excess belly fat, fatigue, acne, loss of libido, foggy thinking, depression, excessive weeping, bloating, and headaches in both genders. It can also cause PMS, irregular periods, endometriosis and fibrocystic or swollen breasts in women.

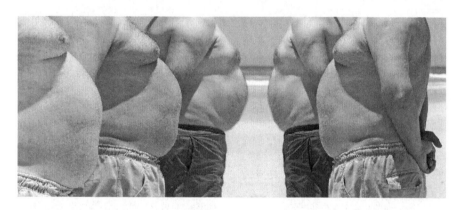

Certain forms of estrogen are potent suppressors of testosterone, and the more estrogen you have in your system, the less testosterone you will have available to pump up your sex drive. Estrogen dominance can take away from a man's masculinity by causing muscle and hair loss, and the development of fatty tissue in the breasts, or "man boobs." It can also cause a reduced ability to achieve erections, lower sperm count, difficult urination, heightened emotional sensitivity, infertility, and premature/rapid ejaculation. I've had countless patients tell me they have stronger, longer lasting erections (improving from three minutes to 20+) and ejaculate with greater force and intensity after lowering estrogen and optimizing testosterone and DHT levels.

Worth noting, there is a cyclical link where weight gain leads to estrogen dominance and estrogen dominance leads to weight gain. This is fueled by aromatase which is an enzyme that converts testosterone into a potent type of estrogen called estradiol. Aromatase is stored in fat cells, and an increase in fat cells leads to higher aromatase and thus higher estrogen levels. Unfortunately, an increase in estrogen also causes an increase in weight gain because it leads to a loss of muscle mass, and consequently a lowered metabolism. Estrogen dominance also contributes to insulin insensitivity. This encourages weight gain because an insensitivity to insulin reduces the ability of the cells to usher glucose to the liver and muscles, which results in higher blood glucose levels, and the excess glucose is stored as fat. Losing excess body weight is thus an essential step for reversing estrogen dominance.

Another major cause of estrogen dominance is birth control pills. The pill is problematic because it introduces excessive amounts of the extremely potent type of estrogen called estradiol into the body. Birth control pills also increase sex-hormone-binding-globulin (SHBG) which lowers testosterone levels, and these hormonal changes often lead to a loss of sex drive and numerous other sexual side-effects. If you want a safe alternative to the birth control pill, consider using condoms, or combining the withdrawal method (don't use this on its own) with fertility awareness. There are plenty of apps available to help you with fertility awareness, but

Natural Cycles is the only one that is certified for contraception.

The diet and lifestyle modifications recommended throughout this book will help to lower estrogen levels. Make sure to include plenty of cruciferous veggies as well because they are the richest sources of the phytonutrients -- DIM and I3C, and these two nutrients have a uniquely powerful ability to remove estrogens from your body.

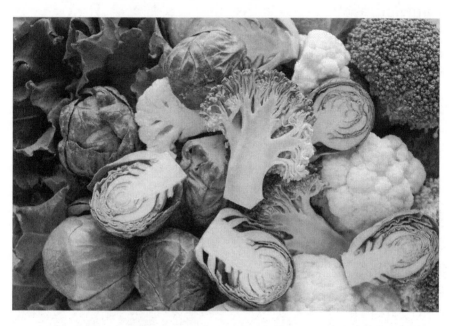

You should also consume a fiber-rich diet and reduce your exposure to xenoestrogens by eating organic, whole foods, replacing plastic food and beverage containers with glass, using organic cleaning and personal care products, and sweating frequently with exercise and saunas (so long as you're not a male who is struggling with infertility, in which case avoid the sauna).

The above recommendations will definitely reduce toxic estrogens, but they are rarely powerful enough on their own to reverse estrogen dominance once it has fully developed. For added support, I recommend you take a nutraceutical that contains concentrated doses of DIM and I3C, such as EstroBlock, in combination with Neuro Insight, which aids in the clearing of the estrogens that exert the most toxic effects in the body. If you're overweight or your estradiol levels are notably elevated, you may also want to take Liv D-Tox because a healthy liver dramatically increases the metabolism and elimination of toxic estrogens.

How to Increase Estrogen Levels

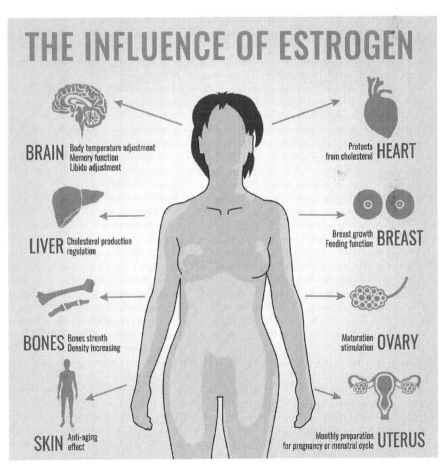

An estrogen deficiency can occur in men (especially if they are using testosterone replacement therapy without proper monitoring); however, it is far more common in women. It is frequently found in premenopausal and menopausal women and in women who exercise excessively, have eating disorders, or who have extremely low body fat. Low estrogen can lead to reduced lubrication and painful sex, infertility, lethargy, and mood swings in women, and increased body fat, fatigue, oversleeping, irritability, loss of libido, reduced fertility, and erectile dysfunction in men.[66] [67]

You can boost estrogen by consuming organic, whole-food soy products (edamame, tempeh, miso, tofu etc.) and other foods that are high in plant-based estrogens (phytoestrogens), such as legumes, flax seeds, licorice, wheat berries, oats, barley, and green and red clover tea. Herbal supplements such as Chastetree berry (make sure to monitor testosterone levels if you use this because it can cause a deficiency) and Dong Quai can also help. If these things fail to restore your estrogen to healthy levels, have a functional medicine practitioner write a bioidentical hormone replacement therapy (BHRT) prescription for you.

How to Increase Testosterone

As I've stated throughout the book, testosterone plays a leading role in sexual health and is essential for sexual desire, arousal and pleasure in both males and females. For my female readers, if you have ever wondered why men are so hyper-focused on sex, the answer is testosterone. Most men

---

[66] http://www.endocrine-abstracts.org/ea/0020/ea0020s4.4.htm
[67] https://www.renalandurologynews.com/hypogonadism/low-estrogen-explains-some-hypogonadal-symptoms-in-men/article/311348/

have an average of ten times more testosterone than women. Unfortunately, testosterone progressively declines after the age of 20 in both genders. To make matters worse, sex-hormone-binding-globulin (SHBG) often increases with age, which binds to testosterone and renders it useless. And aromatization (the conversion of testosterone into estrogen) tends to increase with age as well, which further reduces testosterone levels.

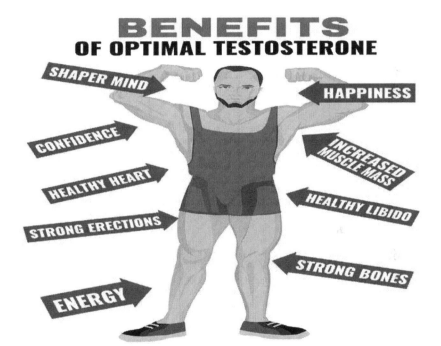

In addition to aging, other possible causes of low testosterone include trauma, steroid use, genetic disorders, radiation, and illnesses such as diabetes, liver disease, COPD, HIV, pituitary gland disorders, and kidney disease. Common testosterone deficiency symptoms that are experienced by both genders include a reduced sex drive, loss of libido, delayed or weak orgasms, excess belly fat, muscle loss, inability to lose weight, low mood, and lethargy. Women may also experience vaginal dryness and painful sex, and men may experience reduced sperm volume, weaker erections, and problems with conception (it's estimated that the male plays a role in a quarter to a half of all couples with fertility problems).

If you experience deficiency symptoms, have your testosterone levels measured. But listen up: many conventional doctors base their diagnoses on "total" testosterone levels, but even if your total levels are high, you can suffer deficiency symptoms if you don't have enough "free" testosterone or if you have too much estrogen. Make sure they test your estrogen and your free testosterone levels. You may also experience symptoms if your levels are on the low-end of normal, so be sure to keep that in mind when assessing your test results.

You can purchase an extremely accurate 24-hour urine kit that tests for free and total testosterone, five estrogens, and all of the other key hormones that affect sexual health here: https://delgadoprotocol.com/product/24-hour-urine-analysis/. Or purchase a saliva panel test (which is less costly) and measures 11 key hormones here: https://delgadoprotocol.com/product/11-hormone-saliva-panel/

Testosterone Replacement Therapy (TRT) is a common solution for low testosterone levels. However, TRT often worsens estrogen dominance because as mentioned above, the aromatase enzyme converts testosterone into estrogen. Unfortunately, most men aren't aware of this, and some attempt to fix their estrogen dominance symptoms by taking more testosterone, which worsens their condition.

Fortunately, you can boost testosterone without causing estrogen dominance with natural techniques. Start by reducing xenoestrogen exposure, having more sex, and incorporating the diet and exercise recommendations provided in this book. You should also optimize your vitamin D levels (vitamin D plays a role in testosterone production) by either exposing your skin to 15 minutes of sunlight a day, or by taking a vitamin D3 pill.

Herbs and nutraceuticals are also extremely effective at restoring youthful testosterone levels for both men and women. Tongkat Ali is particularly beneficial and clinically proven to increase testosterone levels and reduce sex-hormone-binding-globulin (SHBG).[68] Other beneficial herbs include Maca, Tribulus terrestris, Avena sativa, and stinging nettles.[69] These herbs increase free testosterone levels by preventing SHBG from binding to it.

TestroVida Pro contains Tongkat Ali in a concentrated dose of 200:1, which makes it much more effective than other supplements that provide it in lower concentrations. It also contains all the above-mentioned testosterone boosting herbs, plus adaptogens (which indirectly boost testosterone by helping to reduce stress), and zinc which is essential for the production of testosterone.

Testrogenesis cream (see appendix) can also produce amazing results in both women and men. It contains a natural androgen called Laxogenin that a research friend of mine, Mike Mahler, suggested I look into. When I read the research and then tried this natural booster for myself, I was astonished by its libido-enhancing powers. This product contains

---

[68] https://www.hindawi.com/journals/ecam/2012/818072/
[69] https://www.ncbi.nlm.nih.gov/pmc/articles/PMC4120469/

pregnenolone and DHEA, hormones that decline naturally with age and that many adults are deficient in. DHEA is a precursor to testosterone and helps to optimize its production. The pregnenolone helps to boost testosterone along with a range of herbs that reduce toxic estrogens and aid in reversing sexual dysfunction. Using a cream is beneficial because it is absorbed from your skin directly into your bloodstream, bypassing the need for proper digestion and absorption.

If you have a severe testosterone deficiency, you may want to consider bioidentical hormone replacement therapy (BHRT). Testosterone pellets which are implanted under the skin are the ideal delivery method because they mimic the body exactly and release testosterone in much smaller amounts throughout the day, which reduces side-effects and its conversion to estrogen.

Chapter 7
Reversing Sexual Dysfunction and Infertility and Maximizing Libido

Optimizing hormone and neurotransmitter levels is vitally important for your physical, emotional, sexual and relational health, but for optimal benefits, the following guidelines should also be adhered to.

Exercise Regularly

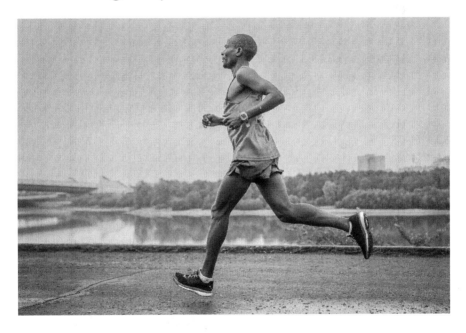

Regular exercise enhances your sexual health in a multitude of ways, and research shows sexual satisfaction progressively increases as fitness levels improve. Exercise makes you feel more confident and sexier, it enhances libido, it helps to lower artery-clogging cholesterol, it increases nitric oxide (and clitoral and penile blood flow), and it reduces the risk for ED. It also helps to boost testosterone which, as has been stated, is the most important hormone for sexual desire and function. Plus, it fights stress, depression, and anxiety -- three of the leading psychological saboteurs of sex. And because it increases strength and endurance, it can help you perform better between the sheets.

Your exercise regime should include a combination of cardiovascular, strength training, and flexibility building exercises. Try to get at least 300 minutes of cardio a week. High intensity interval training (HIIT) is an excellent form of cardio that will bring greater results in shorter periods of time. Strength training exercises should also be done at least three times a week. You may also want to include exercises that strengthen the shoulders, chest, and abs (push-ups, sit-ups, crunches etc.). These are beneficial because building upper body strength will increase your stamina in bed.

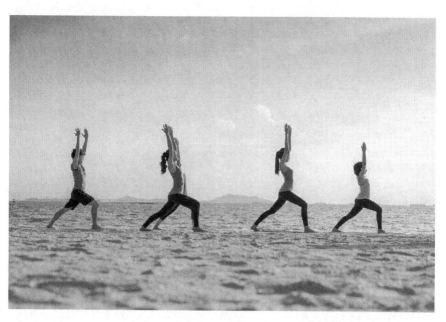

Stretching and deep breathing exercises are also essential and should be included at a bare minimum, twice a week. If you want to experience better sex, then erotic yoga (taught in San Francisco by my friend Brett at a club called Twist) is arguably the best way to incorporate your stretching and deep breathing exercises. Any type of yoga will do however; the practice itself is sensual in nature, and helps bring awareness to sensations in the body, increases pelvic floor muscles, helps heal mental blocks to sexual health, and can enhance desire, arousal, and orgasmic intensity. Plus, you may pick-up some ideas for new sex positions in the process!

One final type of exercise I recommend is rebounding with a trampoline. Ten minutes a day will help enhance the lymph system and remove toxins that can cause fatigue and lethargy. It will also dramatically enhance blood circulation and pelvic floor strength. For the best exercise and diet tips take our online   course: https://delgadoprotocol.com/modules/persistent-weight-loss/

Enhance Arterial Health

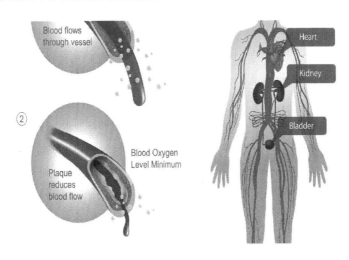

As mentioned earlier, arterial health is required for the flow of blood to the sexual pleasure organs. The best way to enhance heart health and prevent/reverse clogged arteries is to consume the diet laid-out in Chapter 9. Aim for a minimum of 70 grams of fiber a day (or take soluble fibers), exercise regularly, boost nitric oxide, reduce alcohol and stress, and stop smoking. For added support you can also take PCOS Heart Plus (see appendix)-- it contains a variety of nutrients that help to lower cholesterol levels and enhance heart health.

Perform Kegels

Aging, excess body weight, pregnancy, childbirth, and surgery can weaken pelvic floor muscles in both genders.[70] Kegel exercises can help strengthen and tighten those muscles and make sex more pleasurable for you and your partner. Kegels enhance blood flow to the penis, clitoris, and vagina, and by strengthening the pelvic muscles that contract during orgasm, they can make your orgasms more intense and easier to achieve. They can also help relieve certain types of female sexual pain because they teach a woman how to control the pelvic floor muscles so that she can relax them during intercourse.

Actively Detox

Our bodies have powerful detoxifying capabilities, but they were not designed to deal with the slew of modern-day toxins (processed foods, heavy metals, PCBs, endocrine disruptors, chemical toxins in personal care products, etc.) that we currently encounter. Our livers can easily become

---

[70] https://www.mayoclinic.org/healthy-lifestyle/mens-health/in-depth/kegel-exercises-for-men/art-20045074

overwhelmed by all these toxins, and when the liver is unable to keep up, several hormone imbalances can develop.[71]

We need to help reduce the burden on our livers and eliminative organs by reducing the amount of toxins we introduce into our bodies. Eliminate or vastly reduce your intake of sugar, alcohol, nicotine, and caffeine, and reduce your exposure to environmental estrogen-like compounds (xenoestrogens) by drinking and showering in filtered water and using organic cleaning and personal care products. You should also eliminate or limit your intake of fish, especially the larger ones such as tuna and salmon, because they are concentrated sources of toxic heavy metals. If you do eat fish, scallops, sole, and halibut are healthier options.

Staying properly hydrated is also helpful. An easy way to monitor your hydration status is to look at your urine - it should be clear and not yellow. Sweating with saunas and intense exercise is also beneficial. For a more pronounced detoxification effect, I recommend you take Liv D-Tox, which contains the ultimate liver supporting herb Silymarin, and a blend of other regenerative herbs (see appendix).

Make Frequent Sex a Priority

One of the best ways to enhance sexual desire and satisfaction is to have more sex. Having sex helps to naturally increase testosterone levels, oxytocin, and other feel-good hormones and chemicals -- all of which enhance libido. Studies show the more frequently a woman has sex, the more quickly and easily she will become aroused. A high frequency of sex also lowers the risk of cardiovascular events for both

---

[71] https://www.womensinternational.com/portfolio-items/liver/

genders, and the risk for ED in men.[72] Consider enjoying early morning sex, as this is the time a man's testosterone and HGH is at its highest and his erection the firmest, which can make sex more pleasurable for both of you!

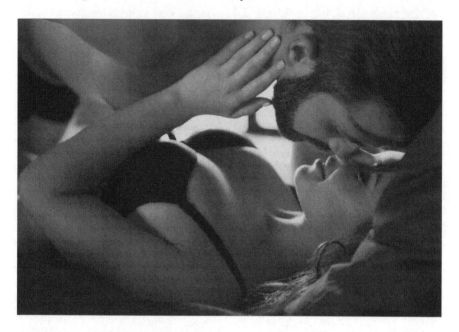

Take Nutraceuticals

Many of my clients who suffer with poor libido and arousal, and/or premature ejaculation, have experienced great success by taking Liv D-Tox in combination with either DHT Block or EstroBlock. This combination helps to maximize the removal of toxic estrogens from the body (see Chapter 6), including estrogens that are stored in fat cells. After taking these supplements for a few weeks, I then have them add Neuro Insight which aids in the clearing of the estrogens that exert the most toxic effects in the body. As an added benefit, this protocol which excretes toxic estrogens may also help

---

[72] https://www.ncbi.nlm.nih.gov/pmc/articles/PMC5052677/

reduce the risk for breast, uterine, and endometrial cancer in women, and shrink an enlarged prostate, and lower the risk for BPH and prostate cancer in men.[73] *see appendix for more on these nutraceuticals

To Reverse Male Infertility

All of the recommendations in this chapter are important for reversing fertility issues in both genders. But men, if you struggle with infertility, you should also avoid heat by switching to boxers, not overdoing it in the sauna, steering clear of overly tight pants, and never putting the laptop on your lap. These recommendations are important because heat interferes with the sperm production process. Losing excess body weight is also important if you struggle with infertility because excess weight leads to extra scrotum fat, which increases the temperature of your sperm, killing and immobilizing them in the process.

Stress is another proven fertility killer. You should actively reduce it with things such as meditation, deep breathing, yoga, journaling, being in nature, and proper time management. I also recommend you have your prolactin levels measured because elevated prolactin is a very common cause of infertility in men. Finally, avoid alcohol, soda, soy (it appears to reduce sperm count), and marijuana (it reduces erectile strength). And consider taking CoQ10, ginseng, Eurycoma Longifolia, and/or l-arginine supplements. Dietary modifications are also an essential step in reversing sexual dysfunction, and we will explore the ideal diet in Chapter 9.

---

[73] http://www.cumc.columbia.edu/publications/in-vivo/Vol2_Iss10_may26_03/

5

Chapter 8
Safe and Effective Ways to Reverse Premature Ejaculation

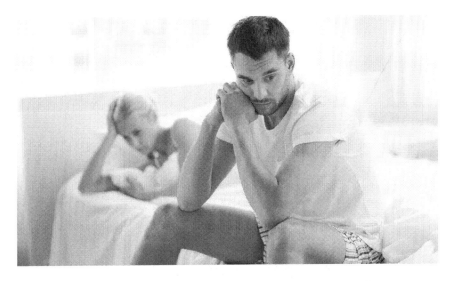

Premature ejaculation, or PE, is the term for a man ejaculating sooner during sexual intercourse than he or his partner would like. Premature ejaculation can be caused by psychological and biological factors, and it is the most common form of sexual dysfunction. It affects one in three men, it is almost always treatable, and it is nothing to be embarrassed about. Below is an outline of safe and effective ways to reverse PE. Often a blend of different therapies will produce the greatest benefit, and your course of treatment should be personalized to address the underlying cause of your PE.

Diagnosing PE

When PE happens infrequently, it is not considered a true sexual dysfunction, and it's nothing to be concerned about. In order to be diagnosed with premature ejaculation, you need to meet the following three criteria, provided by Mayo Clinic:[74]

1. You always or almost always ejaculate within one minute of penetration
2. You're incapable of delaying ejaculation during intercourse all or nearly all the time
3. You feel frustration and distress and tend to avoid sexual intimacy as a result

Treatment Options for PE:

Psychological-Behavioral Therapy

Premature ejaculation is often caused by stress or performance anxiety. Addressing these psychological causes may be all that is required to reverse it, especially in younger men.[75] According to Michael Castleman, M.A.: "In our culture, men are supposed to orchestrate sex, but few young men know much about lovemaking. This causes anxiety, which makes the nervous system more excitable and more prone to PE, which often becomes a conditioned reflex that can last a lifetime".[76]

Fortunately, there is a simple solution – shift the focus away from the genitals and intercourse and do the opposite of

---

[74] https://www.mayoclinic.org/diseases-conditions/premature-ejaculation/symptoms-causes/syc-20354900
[75] https://www.psychologytoday.com/us/blog/all-about-sex/201005/premature-ejaculation-the-two-causes-mens-1-sex-problem
[76] https://www.psychologytoday.com/us/blog/all-about-sex/201005/premature-ejaculation-the-two-causes-mens-1-sex-problem

what you see in porn. Practice deep breathing and relaxation, and engage in long, sensual, massage-based foreplay, which will take pressure off the penis. Practicing tantric sex can also be tremendously helpful (to learn more refer to Chapter 15). If the above fails and you believe there are deeper rooted psychological factors at play, consider NLP, hypnotherapy, cognitive behavioral therapy, or counselling.

The Pause-Squeeze Technique

The pause-squeeze technique is beneficial for many PE sufferers. Start foreplay and include penile stimulation until you feel like you're almost ready to ejaculate. Then have your partner squeeze the point on your penis where the head joins the shaft for several seconds, until your urge to ejaculate subsides.[77] Repeat this process as often as is necessary, and you may eventually reach the point where you can enter your partner without climaxing. According to Mayo Clinic, practicing this several times may make the feeling of knowing how to delay ejaculation a habit that no longer requires the use of this technique.[78]

Additional Sexual Techniques

Some men benefit by masturbating an hour or two before they plan to have sex.[79] This technique is not ideal for most older men however, because the refractory period often lengthens with age, so it can cause difficulties with erection

---

[77] https://www.mayoclinic.org/diseases-conditions/premature-ejaculation/diagnosis-treatment/drc-20354905
[78] https://www.mayoclinic.org/diseases-conditions/premature-ejaculation/diagnosis-treatment/drc-20354905
[79] https://www.mayoclinic.org/diseases-conditions/premature-ejaculation/diagnosis-treatment/drc-20354905

and ejaculation during sex. Another technique is to stop all sexual activity right before you ejaculate and wait until you've cooled down before proceeding again. Using thick condoms can also be beneficial because they reduce the sensitivity of the penis; you can even purchase "climax control" condoms over the counter. Applying a numbing cream or spray, such as lidocaine or benzocaine, 10 to 15 minutes before sex may also help, states Mayo Clinic.[80]

Pelvic Exercises

Weak pelvic floor muscles can impair the ability to delay ejaculation; you can use pelvic exercises (Kegels) to strengthen these muscles. To identify the correct muscles, stop urination in midstream. Tighten these muscles, hold for three seconds, and then release for three seconds. Repeat this exercise ten times to complete a set and aim for three sets a day.[81] You can do these exercises sitting, standing, walking, or lying down.

Herbal Therapy

Although no scientific studies have been conducted to prove this discovery, I found in my clinic that a combination of highly concentrated herbs including turmeric, astragalus, and asparagus delayed ejaculation from the normal three minutes to thirty minutes. Liv D-Tox has these necessary herbs, and I typically combine it with EstroBlock and Neuro Insight to reverse premature ejaculation caused by estrogen dominance.

---

[80] https://www.mayoclinic.org/diseases-conditions/premature-ejaculation/diagnosis-treatment/drc-20354905
[81] https://www.mayoclinic.org/diseases-conditions/premature-ejaculation/diagnosis-treatment/drc-20354905

Korean ginseng berry may also be beneficial. Ginseng is a popular herb in Traditional Chinese Medicine for the treatment of all types of sexual dysfunction, and a study published in the *International Journal of Impotence Research* found 1.4 g of Korean ginseng berry extract taken daily for 4 weeks, significantly improved PE.[82]

5-HTP

Although 5-HTP is not clinically proven for the treatment of PE, it is well documented in medical literature to produce similar effects as antidepressant medications. Antidepressants are the classical treatment for PE by allopathic doctors.[83] [84] 5-HTP may help with premature ejaculation by increasing serotonin levels, and while it may not be powerful enough to stop PE completely, it may at least slow the process, states Ray Sahelian, M.D..[85]

Hormone Therapy

The following recommendations from Dr. Thierry Hertoghe only apply if your premature ejaculation is caused by the fact that you cannot hold an erection very long (another type of sexual dysfunction), so you rush to orgasm out of anxiety. Low testosterone is a major cause of sexual dysfunction and an inability to maintain an erection. If a total and free testosterone test indicate low testosterone, optimizing it with an herbal supplement (see appendix) may help

---

[82] https://www.nature.com/articles/ijir201245
[83] https://www.asianjournalofpsychiatry.com/article/S1876-2018(12)00117-7/fulltext
[84] https://www.mayoclinic.org/diseases-conditions/premature-ejaculation/diagnosis-treatment/drc-20354905
[85] http://www.raysahelian.com/prematureejaculation.html

enhance erection longevity, so you no longer rush to ejaculation. DHEA may also help because it is a precursor hormone that turns into several important sex hormones including testosterone.[86] You can boost DHEA safely and optimize sex hormone balance with Testro Vida Cream.

And finally, if all else fails, you may want to try Melanotan II injections.[87] This injection is administered under the skin near your belly with a protein peptide also referred to as Bremelanotide PT-141. The fantasy center of the brain seems involved with this potent libido and powerful erectile function protein. Be aware these injections may increase the tan pigments (melanin) and cause skin darkening. I told my friend Ron Rothenberg, MD, an expert in hormone replacement about PT-141, and a few years later he showed up at an anti-aging conference with a deep rich tan and smiled telling me my suggestion was absolutely correct: "The use of PT-141 about one hour prior to intimacy is an amazing enhancer of sexual function."

---

[86] https://www.ncbi.nlm.nih.gov/pubmed/10096389

[87] https://www.semanticscholar.org/paper/Melanocortin-receptor-agonists%2C-penile-erection%2C-II-Wessells-Levine/057a269abc828b59aabc2de20f2c243b8fb11f72

Chapter 9
The Sexual Health and Libido-Boosting Diet

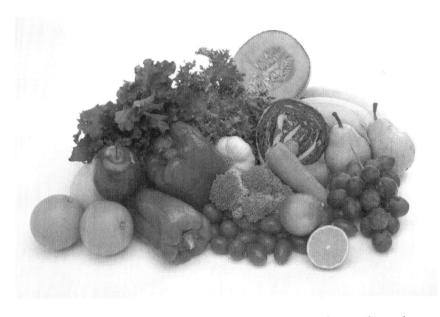

Many people falsely associate meat with virility, but a whole-foods, plant-based diet is by far the most effective way to maximize sexual health, function, and pleasure. Meat and dairy are problematic because they are major contributors to estrogen dominance. In fact, animal products are the highest dietary sources of estrogen, and factory farming practices make the estrogen load even higher because many animals are injected with estradiol (an estrogen metabolite) in order to enhance their growth.[88] [89] [90]

---

[88] https://www.youtube.com/watch?v=zLENOIB4wEs
[89] https://www.ncbi.nlm.nih.gov/pmc/articles/PMC3834504/

Dairy products are the absolute worst offenders. Researchers have found that milk makes up 60-70% of the total estrogen consumed in the average American diet.[91] Plus every time you consume animal products, their fat content increases your triglyceride levels, which accelerates the clogging of your arteries and reduces pleasurable blood flow to your sexual organs. Researchers have found a plant-based diet has the added benefit of increasing testosterone levels.[92]

Sugar and vegetable oils are highly inflammatory; they elevate triglycerides and should be eliminated as well. If completely eliminating these foods is unfeasible for you, then limit your intake as much as possible. Repetitively consuming these products leads to chronically elevated triglyceride levels which accelerates the artery-clogging process. This is made even worse if you smoke cigarettes because carbon monoxide in the smoke combines with oxygen nearly 200 times more powerfully, reducing your red blood cells' ability to transport oxygen throughout the body. Note: I suggest you use whole olives in place of olive oil or edamame in place of soy oil.

A low-fat diet comprised primarily of vegetables and fruits, as well as beans, legumes, and rice, will enhance physical appearance, improve hormones, release youth-enhancing peptides, and significantly improve sexual desire and function. Vegans also smell and taste better which makes love making more pleasing for your partner. Emphasizing foods that are high in zinc and B vitamins is also

---

[90]

https://lawpublications.barry.edu/cgi/viewcontent.cgi?article=1001&context=facultyscholarship

[91] https://www.ncbi.nlm.nih.gov/pmc/articles/PMC4524299/

[92] https://nutritionfacts.org/2013/02/12/less-cancer-in-vegan-men-despite-more-testosterone/

recommended to help optimize testosterone levels. Some of the richest plant-based sources of B-vitamins include brewer's yeast, lentils, black beans, pine nuts, spinach, mushrooms, and sunflower seeds. Zinc-rich plant foods include pomegranates, berries, pumpkin seeds, beans, legumes, potatoes, pumpkin and avocados.

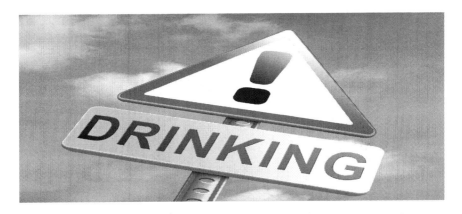

It is also important to limit or eliminate alcohol. Alcohol reduces lubrication and clitoral sensitivity in females, and it is a major cause of erectile dysfunction in men (studies show the more that is consumed, the greater the ED risk).[93] Alcohol use negatively affects all three parts of the hypothalamic-pituitary-gonadal (HPG) axis, which is a system of endocrine glands and hormones involved in male sexual functioning.[94] Alcohol is also produced with plants that contain estrogen-like compounds (phytoestrogens) which can worsen estrogen dominance in men and women.

If you want to learn how to make delicious, satisfying and easy recipes that adhere to these dietary guidelines, get a copy of the *Simply Healthy - The Delgado Diet Cookbook*. The book

---

[93] https://www.ncbi.nlm.nih.gov/pmc/articles/PMC2917074/
[94] https://pubs.niaaa.nih.gov/publications/arh25-4/282-287.htm

includes over 300 recipes with cuisines from around the world that are ideally balanced in protein, whole superfood complex carbohydrates, and essential fats from whole foods to optimize hormone balance, circulation, and sexual functioning.

List of Recommended Foods and Foods to Avoid

Fruits

Recommended: Any fresh, or unsweetened, frozen or water-packed fruits

Avoid: Dried fruits (small servings without added sugars may be okay if you don't have blood sugar imbalances), and canned, sweetened fruits

Vegetables

Recommended: All fresh raw, steamed, sautéed, juiced, or roasted vegetables

Avoid: Corn and creamed vegetables that have added sugar or milk

Starches

Recommended: Complex unprocessed fiber, starches, e.g. brown rice, oats, millet, quinoa, potato flour, arrowroot, amaranth, tapioca, buckwheat, potatoes

Avoid: Wheat, corn, all gluten-containing products, breads, breakfast cereals, and products made from wheat or containing yeast

Legumes

Recommended: All legumes including peas and lentils

Avoid: Tofu, soybeans, soy milk, and other soy products (organic, fermented soy in moderation may be okay for certain individuals who do not have high estrogen levels)

Nuts and Seeds

Recommended: Almonds, cashews, pecans, walnuts, sesame (tahini), sunflower, pumpkin, and all nut butters (except peanut)

Avoid: Peanuts and peanut butter

Dairy and Milk Substitutes

Recommended: Almond milk, rice milk, hemp milk, coconut milk and all other nut milks

Avoid: Cow's and goat's milk, cheese, cottage cheese, yogurt, butter, ice cream, frozen yogurt, eggs, non-dairy creamers and soy milk

Fats

Recommended: Avocados, seeds, safflower, walnuts, almonds, grape seed, olives, coconuts

Avoid: Processed and hydrogenated oils, all vegetable oils, margarine, butter, shortening, mayonnaise, spreads, poultry skin, deep fried foods, chips, donuts

Beverages

Recommended: Filtered or distilled PH balanced water, unsweetened coconut water, herbal tea, seltzer or mineral water

Avoid: Sodas, diet sodas, sports beverages, and other soft drinks and mixes, alcoholic beverages, coffee, tea, or other caffeinated beverages

Spices and Condiments

Recommended: Vinegar (except malt), raw apple cider vinegar (in abundance); all spices including salt, pepper, cinnamon, cumin, dill, garlic, ginger, carob, oregano, parsley, dry mustard, rosemary, tarragon, thyme or turmeric

Avoid: Ketchup, chutney, BBQ sauce, bottled mustard, and other condiments

Sweeteners

Recommended: Lo Han Guo and stevia, agave nectar, brown rice syrup, fruit sweeteners, and blackstrap molasses (in moderation to avoid blood sugar fluctuations)

Avoid: White or brown refined sugar, artificial sweeteners (aspartame, sweet-n-low etc.), honey, maple syrup, corn syrup, high fructose corn syrup, and evaporated cane sugar

Additional Foods to Avoid:

Processed foods containing baking soda or cornstarch, processed starch foods containing any of the ingredients or sweeteners to avoid

Part 3
Guidelines for Maximizing Pleasure and Becoming an Amazing Lover

Chapter 10
Female Orgasm Inhibitors

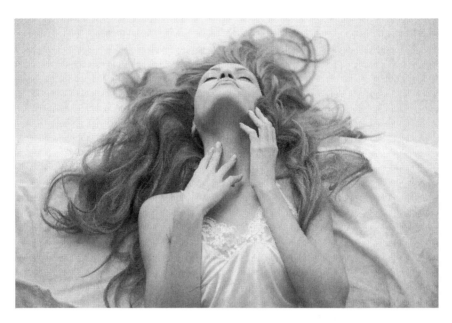

In the beginning of this book I mentioned that a mere 30% of women report having an orgasm every time, and 67% of them admit to faking it (either to end the act more quickly or to spare their partner's feelings). Yet men report having orgasms in approximately 95% of their sexual encounters. Perhaps even more saddening is the fact that 10% to 15% of women never climax under any circumstance, and 72% of women report being with a partner who climaxed but didn't attempt to help them do the same.[95] There is clearly something wrong here, and we will explore the biggest culprits below.

---

[95] https://www.psychologytoday.com/blog/all-about-sex/200903/the-most-important-sexual-statistic

The Biggest Female Orgasm Inhibitors

Female Orgasm Inhibitor #1 - The Vaginal Orgasm Myth

This biggest inhibitor to the female orgasm is the misconception that vaginal intercourse alone should lead to sexual climax. This is untrue for approximately 98% of the female population. It can make a woman feel like there is something wrong with her and put pressure on her to achieve something that is physiologically impossible. As for the few women who are able to climax from intercourse, researchers suggest it is because the distance between their clitoris and vagina allows for inadvertent clitoral stimulation during intercourse.

Men, listen up: The vast majority of women require direct clitoral stimulation to experience orgasm. This is because the pleasure nerve endings are concentrated and attached to the clitoris, and the interior walls of the vagina have very few nerve endings (aside from the g-spot, which is actually an internal extension of the clitoris). This is why size and girth don't matter, and why "going deep" does not equate to greater pleasure for women.

If the male partner fails to provide clitoral stimulation, the female partner will likely be left unsatisfied. The reduced desire to engage in sex that can result from being left unsatisfied can cause her man to feel sex-starved, and a vicious cycle can be created, resulting in either lifelong sexual dissatisfaction between both partners or separation.

Female Orgasm Inhibitor #2 - The Time Discrepancy

Another inhibitor of the female orgasm is the time discrepancy that exists between men and women for reaching orgasm. The average man takes less than two minutes, whereas the average woman requires a bare minimum of twenty minutes and sometimes up to an hour in order to get worked up enough to climax. The solution to this problem is for the man to spend a significant amount of time pleasuring his woman and making sure she is fully worked up before initiating intercourse. And cunnilingus prior to intercourse should be the rule, not the exception, because oral sex is the most effective way for a woman to achieve orgasm.

Female Orgasm Inhibitor #3 - Lack of Foreplay

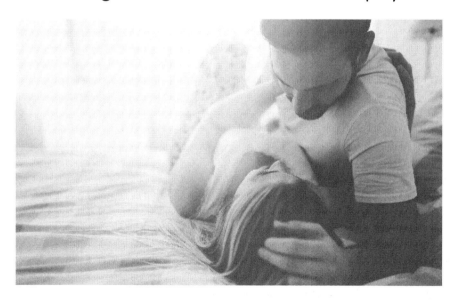

Foreplay is way too short in most sexual encounters, and sometimes it is skipped altogether. When couples jump straight to penetration, the man is often left satisfied, but the woman is not. Men, if you care about your woman and want to be an unselfish lover, then you need to dedicate (with enthusiasm) as much time and energy as she requires in the foreplay stage. And foreplay doesn't mean immediately reaching for the genitals or breasts - you should slowly build-up tension and desire in your women by exploring her entire body and teasing her for at least five minutes before you go near her sexual organs.

Female Orgasm Inhibitor #4 - Focusing Only on Touch

Women require more than just physical stimulation in order to become aroused and to reach orgasm. Female pleasure starts with the brain. Words can have a powerful effect on arousal, and they can be used inside and outside the bedroom. Open communication before, during, and after sex is also important. Communicate openly with each other without judgment, and women, don't be afraid to tell your man what turns you on and share your sexual fantasies. This will eliminate the guesswork of knowing how to please you, and your man will appreciate that as much as you will.

Men, you should alleviate any anxiety that your woman may have about receiving oral sex by telling her how much you love it, how it gets you off, and how her taste turns you on. Compliment her often and make her feel good about her achievements, as well as her body and appearance. I also recommend you and your partner familiarize yourselves with *The 5 Love Languages*. Learning how each of you gives and receives love will strengthen your emotional and spiritual bond, and the positive changes will translate to the bedroom.

Female Orgasm Inhibitor #5 - Attitudes and Thoughts on Sex

Some women were taught to perceive sex as immoral or bad, some have a fear of being vulnerable or losing control, and some have a fear of arousing repressed memories of abuse and trauma.[96] Many women also find it hard to let go and get out of their heads and into their bodies. Some feel guilty about receiving pleasure and taking "too long" to reach orgasm when their man is giving them oral stimulation. And sadly, the vast majority of women have body image issues.

Regardless of your gender, if you have sexual inhibitions or other psychological inhibitors that are preventing you from climaxing or receiving the pleasure that you deserve, you may want to consider Time-Line Therapy, self-hypnosis, CBT, and/or LFC glasses (with audio files for optimal sex, such as: https://delgadoprotocol.com/product/lfc-audio-love-your-body/). These scripts on can be downloaded to your phone or ipad and listened to prior to sex to help overcome subconscious and conscious blocks.

Female Orgasm Inhibitors #6 - Porn Films

Too many men model their sexual behavior off what they see on porn. The problem is, most porn is created for men, by men, and foreplay is rushed or non-existent, or it consists of a few seconds of kissing followed by the woman giving the man fellatio. Rarely do you see the man focusing on the woman's pleasure or giving the woman oral sex for more than a few seconds, yet any truly caring and knowledgeable lover

---

[96] https://www.psychologytoday.com/blog/the-human-experience/201404/7-factors-affecting-orgasm-in-women

wouldn't even consider entering his woman before patiently arousing her with oral and manual stimulation.

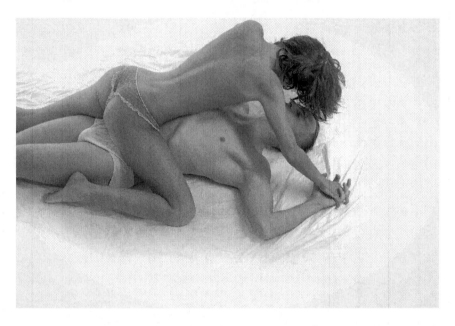

Porn is also problematic because the fast, hard, genital-oriented sex that it glorifies is exactly the opposite of what a woman's body needs. Women are aroused by slow, soft, sensual, whole-body sex. And the importance placed on "size" and "going deep" in porn, and in the media is ridiculous. It is the outer third of the vagina that produces pleasure for a woman and going too deep can actually be painful, especially if you are large, or she is not adequately aroused.

Female Orgasm Inhibitor #7 - Stress

Stress is unavoidable in our modern world, and although it can interfere with pleasure and sexual function in both genders, women are especially impacted by it. An inability to compartmentalize and put stressors aside prevents the relaxation and presence that is required to enjoy sex, and it can make an orgasm nearly impossible.

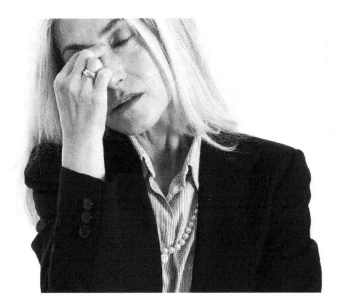

Stress relief techniques before engaging in sex can dramatically improve the entire sexual experience for both genders. Consider yoga, deep breathing exercises, an Epsom salt bath, a massage, meditation, journaling, or anything else that helps you relax. Finally, remember that the way you treat each other outside the bedroom affects your partner's willingness to partake in sex and ability to experience pleasure between the sheets. Keep this in mind if you've been slacking with house chores or other responsibilities that should be shared!

Chapter 11
Advanced Methods to Improve Erections

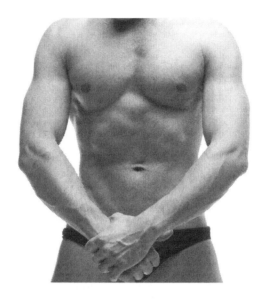

Gentleman, for those of you who enjoy sex and maintaining hard erections, please be aware that the meat, dairy, egg, and processed food-centered diet of the Western world is one of the leading causes of erectile dysfunction (ED). ED is extremely prevalent, and its frequency increases proportionately with age. Approximately 40% of men in their 40s are affected with it, and 70% of men in their 70s.[97]

ED occurs so frequently with age because the arteries to the penis are smaller than the blood vessels to the heart, and blood vessels become restricted and arteries clogged as a

---

[97]
http://www.clevelandclinicmeded.com/medicalpubs/diseasemanagement/endocrinology/erectile-dysfunction/

result of high cholesterol levels which is often caused by animal products.

A diet that is high in animal products is also harmful because it increases prolactin levels, and high levels of prolactin (which acts in a similar manner to estrogen in many ways) is associated with an increased risk for ED. Over 25% of men past the age of 60 who consume unhealthy, high-protein, high-fat diets have ED, while less than 2% have problems while on a plant-based diet. If cleaning up your diet, eliminating alcohol, and implementing the other recommendations in this book fail to reverse your ED, you may want to try the following more advanced methods adjunctively.

PDE5 Inhibitors

As I mentioned earlier in this book, PDE5 inhibitors such as Viagra and Cialis don't work for everyone and often lose their effectiveness with time (because of NO depletion and/or too much plaque build-up). But they are an option, nevertheless. If you take them, I recommend you use them adjunctively with the diet and lifestyle modifications mentioned in this book so that you can reverse the root cause of your ED. Failing to do so will likely result in plaque buildup or NO depletion reaching a point where the medication no longer works, and because lifestyle modifications take time to produce their beneficial effects, you will be out of effective options.

Melanotan II

Melanotan II injections are more potent and effective than Viagra. Melanotan II is a synthetic equivalent of the naturally occurring peptide α-melanocyte-stimulating hormone, or MSH. Its exact mechanism of action has not yet been determined but it appears to work in the brain to stimulate penile erections.[98] Its effects are powerful, and according to the *Journal of Impotence Research,* 17 out of 20 men with erectile dysfunction experienced an erection with Melanotan II without any sexual stimulation.

Melanotan II also increases sexual desire and penile volume, enhances ejaculation, and boosts stamina, producing erections that last approximately 40 minutes.[99] Melanotan II may also produce emotional benefits: studies on animals found it made the animals more affectionate with their partners, reduced quarrelling, and led to quicker mate selection.[100] You can enhance the effectiveness of Melanotan II even further by avoiding alcohol, and in some instances, by combining it with other hormones.[101]

Penile Injectables

Penile injectables can be beneficial when PDE5 inhibitors fail and while waiting for lifestyle modifications to produce their beneficial effects. The idea of injectable medications may sound intimidating and/or painful, but they are actually simple and cause very little discomfort and are considered to be the most powerful class of anti-erectile dysfunction agents. They are injected into the base of the penis with a needle

---

[98] https://www.semanticscholar.org/paper/Melanocortin-receptor-agonists%2C-penile-erection%2C-II-Wessells-Levine/057a269abc828b59aabc2de20f2c243b8fb11f72

[99] https://www.semanticscholar.org/paper/Melanocortin-receptor-agonists%2C-penile-erection%2C-II-Wessells-Levine/057a269abc828b59aabc2de20f2c243b8fb11f72

[100] https://www.youtube.com/watch?v=gNeaPuzxXfl

[101] https://www.youtube.com/watch?v=gNeaPuzxXfl

which can be done at home, and typically produce an erection that lasts up to one hour, within 5 to 20 minutes. Tri-Mix is arguably the most popular injectable; it uses a very tiny needle and it contains a blend of three active ingredients (alprostadil, papaverine, and phentolamine) which act synergistically. Tri-Mix is considered the go-to treatment if a patient is not responsive to Viagra, Cialis or other conventional PDE5 inhibitors.

The Three Active Ingredients in Tri-Mix

Papaverine - Relaxes the smooth muscles and widens the blood vessels (vasodilation) which allows for enhanced blood flow. This ingredient when used alone increases the risk for two penile disorders – priapism and corporal fibrosis; however, this risk is greatly reduced when papaverine is used in very small dosages and combined with alprostadil and phentolamine.

Phentolamine - Causes blood vessels to expand and thereby increases blood flow. It is often combined with papaverine which leads to enhanced efficacy. This combination is supported by substantial clinical research, and one study found the combination yielded a 90% effectiveness rate for producing erections that are sufficient for sexual intercourse.[102]

Prostaglandin E1 or PGE1 (Alprostadil) – Activates prostaglandin receptors (PG) and increases cyclic adenosine monophosphate (cAMP) which leads to smooth muscle relaxation. It is a potent vasodilator and is often combined with papaverine for enhanced efficacy. It is available as a

---

[102] https://www.ncbi.nlm.nih.gov/pubmed/16422914

gel,and as an intraurethral pellet as well; however, it is most effective when injected.[103]

Additional Injectable Ingredients

Atropine – This is sometimes added to Tri-Mix to create a formula referred to as Quad-Mix. It aids in contraction and relaxation of smooth muscles and epithelial tissue in the penis and throughout the body and in the achievement of penile erections. It does this by inhibiting the absorption of a chemical called acetylcholine in penile cells. When used on its own, its efficacy is low. It needs to be combined with other injectables, and the primary benefit of adding atropine is that it helps reduce the pain associated with PGE1 solutions.[104]

Protein Peptides (GHR2 GHR6, Sermorelin) – While not growth hormones themselves, they stimulate the pituitary gland to produce more growth hormones naturally. This is beneficial because growth hormones are thought to enhance sexual performance. Evidence suggests penile erections may be induced by growth hormones through their cGMP stimulating activity on human corpus cavernosum smooth muscle.[105]

PT 141 (Bremelanotide) – A derivative of MSH (melanocyte-stimulating hormones), a hormone that increases sexual arousal and erection firmness. Significant research is

---

[103] Linet OI, Ogrinc FG. Efficacy and safety of intracavernosal alprostadil in men with erectile dysfunction. The Alprostadil Study Group. New England Journal of Medicine. 1996 Apr 4;334(14):873-7

[104] Sogan PR, Teloken C, Souto CA. "Atropine role in the pharmacological erection test: study of 228 patients. Journal of Urology 1997 Nov;158(5):1760-3
[105] https://www.ncbi.nlm.nih.gov/pubmed/11061943

currently being conducted on this peptide for the treatment of low libido and sexual dysfunction.[106]

Shockwave in Combination with PRP

A shockwave machine is a device that was developed to break up kidney stones. It is a painless procedure, and you can use it to release VGED (vascular endothelial growth factor) and grow new blood vessels. Dr. Terry Grossman in Colorado and Michael Grossman, MD, use this in their clinics, then follows it with PRP (platelet rich plasma) injections. PRP is a relatively painless procedure where blood is drawn from the patient, centrifuged to concentrate healing platelets, and then injected back into the site that needs healing. Grossman states that it is not a perfect therapy and doesn't work for everyone, but when it does work, patients are usually extremely happy and experience not only a reversal of ED, but also a notable increase in penile size and girth.[107]

---

[106] https://www.ncbi.nlm.nih.gov/pmc/articles/PMC2694735/
[107] http://www.grossmanwellness.com/our-staff

Chapter 12
Maximizing Her Pleasure (and Giving Her Multiple Orgasms)

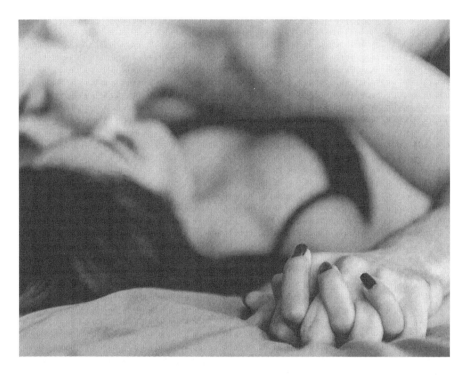

Women deserve orgasms every bit as much as men, and men, it is your job to give it to them! The best way to do so is to learn how to give good oral sex (when done right, nearly 100% of women will achieve orgasm). With the right techniques, you can easily give your women multiple orgasms, and ideally, you should make sure your woman climaxes at least once before entering her. We will explore these techniques later in the chapter but first let's start with some essential steps you need to take outside the bedroom in order to be a truly legendary lover.

Sexual medicine research shows that the motivations for women to have sex are very different than those of men. For men the motivation for sex is rooted in pleasure; it can exist totally independent of a relationship, and it has little to do with emotional intimacy.[108] Women's motivations, on the other hand, center around emotional intimacy; women crave affection, and a genuine, intimate connection.[109] A woman needs to trust you and feel comfortable around you in order to let go and surrender her body fully during sex. And the more emotionally supported and connected she feels to you, the easier it will likely be for her to climax. Women also have greater difficulty getting out of their heads during sex, and if you haven't been treating her right outside of the bedroom, it's going to interfere with her ability to become aroused by you.

If you want your woman to be extremely sexually satisfied, you need to first meet her relationship needs by encouraging her, respecting her, and supporting her. A great way to make her feel emotionally connected to you is by listening to her intently and remembering minute details of what she says. Ask her about her day and pay attention when she mentions liking something; then surprise her by mentioning it or buying it for her weeks later. Do your share of household chores, and surprise her with date nights, a romantic meal at home, thoughtful letters, and flowers or other small gifts that show you are thinking of her.

---

[108] https://www.psychologytoday.com/us/blog/evolution-the-self/201205/the-triggers-sexual-desire-men-vs-women
[109] https://www.psychologytoday.com/us/blog/evolution-the-self/201205/the-triggers-sexual-desire-men-vs-women

Meet her emotional needs by telling her how much you love her and complimenting her often. Build her self-esteem by telling her how sexy she is and how much you love her body. Make sure to compliment her non-sexual attributes as well: tell her how brilliant she is, how beautiful her smile is, how talented she is, how funny she is or whatever it is that you love so much about her.

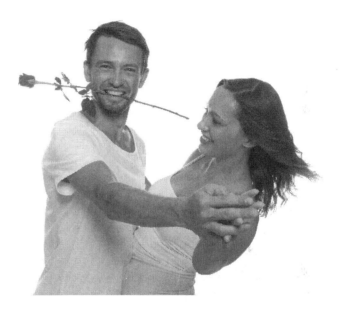

Complimenting her is very important because many women are insecure about their bodies and/or their appearance, and those insecurities can be huge pleasure and orgasm inhibitors. Make her feel cared for any way you can, and don't forget the importance of physical affection. Hold her hand, hug her, snuggle, caress her face and hair, kiss her tenderly, and before initiating sex, give her a sensual massage or a warmed-oil foot rub.

Build her desire and anticipation throughout the day with sexual innuendos and flirty/dirty text messages, notes, or emails. Give her a lingering hug before you leave for work and when you get home and tease her a little bit by pressing your whole body up against her and giving her a sensual kiss. For added provocation, whisper something sexy in her ear such as "I can't wait to rip your clothes off later," or "I've been thinking about your naked body all day." Gently caress her inner thigh when no one is watching and place your hand on her lower back or around her waist while standing next to her.

If you want to boost her sex drive, take stress off her plate wherever you can and make sure to do your share of household and childcare responsibilities. If you have children, after dinner draw her a bath, and tell her you will finish up with the dishes and put the children to bed. Self-care is such a huge, important part of a woman's maintaining of her sexuality, and giving her a little bit of time to care for herself will have a tremendous effect on her mood and sex drive.

You also need to make her feel sexy. Many women get so caught up in the stress of day-to-day living that they completely lose touch with the sexual side of themselves, especially if they have demanding jobs or young children at home. You need to remind your woman how sexy she is, by telling her multiple times, EVERY DAY. Tell her she is the sexiest thing you've ever laid your eyes on, that you can't stop thinking about her, or that she drives you wild, and ogle her blatantly from time-to-time.

Before sex, have a shower and groom yourself diligently. Physical smells are a huge turn-off for women, and if your face is scratchy, your fingernails gnarly, or your genitals unclean or ungroomed, it will distract her from the pleasure she is receiving. Set the physical environment by making sure the temperature is just right and use candles or red-light bulbs to optimize the ambience. If you play music, choose something that turns you both on and set the volume so that it's not too loud or quiet. Lastly, turn off the phone, warm-up some lube and lock the door (if you have children).

How to Send Her Over the Moon with Pleasure (Warning: It's About to Get Graphic)

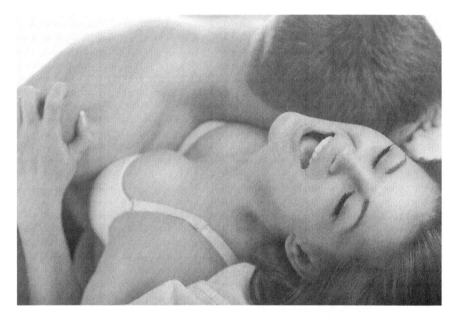

When it is time to get physical, incorporate the motto "foreplay is core-play." Start by touching, caressing, kissing, and licking her entire body. Gently nibble on her neck and forearm, lick in between her thighs, and kiss and suck the skin around her lower belly and hip bone. Slowly work your way to her ears, kiss, nibble and blow gently (if she responds sexually to ear play), and finally make your way to her lips. Passionately kiss her and alternate back and forth from kissing her body to kissing her lips.

Remember that women do not get aroused from visual cues alone, like men do. You need to activate their emotions in order to spark their arousal, and one great way to do that is with your words. For this, the delivery is as important as the words themselves. Say the words in a soft, yet strong and confident tone. If you can whisper them in her ear even better – the feeling of your breath against her ear and neck will add to her arousal. If you don't know what to say, compliments are always good. Choose something that is not generic, sincere, and specific to her – the more special and unique you make her feel, the more aroused she will become. Use the word "you" and "your" often during foreplay and intercourse, such as "You feel/are amazing", "Your kisses make me so hot," "I can't wait to get inside of you," or "You turn me on so much."

Pay close attention to the signals that she is sending (moaning, breathing, tightening of the abdomen, moving her body towards or away from you, and so forth), and when she is clearly worked up, you can make your way to her breasts, and ever so slowly (stopping on the way to kiss and lick her stomach and thighs again) to her outer, and then inner vaginal lips. When she can't take it anymore, move to her clitoris.

Mastering Cunnilingus

If you want to be a legendary lover, it is essential that you understand the clitoris. The clitoral head is the visible part of the clitoris that is protected by the inner lips of the vagina. However, the head is only a tiny part of the clitoris -- more than three quarters of the clitoris is inside a woman's body. "One way I explain the clitoris to both men and women is to understand that the clitoris has legs and these internal legs go into the vagina, bundle at the g-spot, then wave towards the cervix," states sex expert Dr. Dawn Michael.[110] The visible head contains approximately 8,000 nerve endings, which is twice as many as the head of the penis. One of the biggest mistakes a man can make is to underestimate just how sensitive the clitoral head is. Rubbing the head over and over again with the same rhythm and intensity can quickly become irritating. Another common complaint of women is that men are too fast and rough, so be gentle and take it slow.

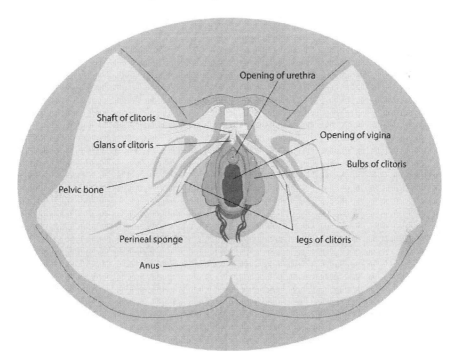

When giving her cunnilingus, consider propping a pillow under her butt. This will help enhance blood flow to her pelvic region, provide you with better access to her genitals, and also help ease tension on your neck. When you stimulate the clitoral head for the first time, press the soft, wet tip of your

[110] https://www.askmen.com/dating/love_tip_200/204_love_tip.html

tongue into it and then hold the position. Next, use rhythmic and gentle tongue strokes and proceed to firmer strokes once arousal levels have increased. According to Ian Kerner, MD, in his book *She Comes First*, cunnilingus is all about the balance between movement and stillness, and you should make sure that the interval between licks is long enough to let each one resonate fully.[111] As she starts to get more worked up, tease her by avoiding the clitoral head and stimulating her labia.

"The best lovers switch it up often, and have a large assortment of techniques in their sexual repertoire" states sex expert and CEO of Personal Life Media (personallifemedia.com), Susan Bratton.[112] They use a variety of licks, sucks and nibbles (soft, hard, wet, fast, intermittent etc.), and stimulate the entire vulva during oral sex. Use your fingers both externally and internally to enhance her pleasure. Slowly insert the first two inches of your index finger inside of her and gently lick her clitoris at the same time. Kerner also advices: "They don't call it giving head for nothing. Cunnilingus involves more than just the use of your tongue. You need to get your whole face in there."[113]

It can take anywhere from 15 to 45 minutes for a woman to reach her first orgasm during cunnilingus, and one of women's largest anxieties is the fear that they are taking too long. So be patient and reassure her by telling her how much you love pleasing her orally. As you become more familiar with her body and she becomes more comfortable with you, the time will often be reduced.

---

[111] https://www.iankerner.com/
[112] www.personallifemedia.com
[113] https://www.amazon.com/She-Comes-First-Thinking-Pleasuring/dp/0060538260

Worth noting: a woman is capable of multiple orgasms, and the time it takes to reach orgasm is often vastly shortened after the first one because her genitals are already engorged, and her body is awash with potent sex chemicals. And a woman's genitals don't become hypersensitive, so with a short break (a few minutes focused on kissing or touching other parts of her body) and a little stimulation, her body is ready to begin the process all over again. Men, on the other hand, have a refractory period that can last between hours and days, and once you enter her, it may not be possible to hold off long enough to bring her to multiple orgasms. So, if you want to be a truly legendary lover, give her the gift of multiple orgasms before proceeding to intercourse.

Mastering Sex

What worked for her last time may not be what she needs this time. Do your homework and constantly collect new techniques so that you will be prepared to adapt to your woman's variable needs. Whatever you do, don't learn your techniques from watching porn. Porn does not teach you how to make love to a woman. Female porn stars screaming in bliss after being penetrated with zero foreplay are simply doing their job -- acting.

For an extremely detailed guide that includes hundreds of techniques for pleasing your woman, including how to find and stimulate her g-spot, I recommend Ian Kerner's New York Time's bestselling book *She Comes First*. Bratton's website, personallifemedia.com, is also loaded with hundreds of detailed techniques and tips for achieving sexual mastery. Study their techniques until they become second nature. This is important because trying to think back and recall different techniques during the moment will make it feel mechanical and take away from both of your pleasure.

Communication is vitally important. Have a talk with her outside the bedroom and let her know that your main goal is to please her. Tell her you want to make sure you are meeting her needs and ask her to give you open and honest feedback in the moment while you are pleasuring her. Tell her she can blurt out whatever comes to mind, that she doesn't have to worry about sugar coating her requests and assure her you will never take offence to her suggestions. When she gives you feedback, say something simple such as "okay baby" and NEVER be defensive or apologetic. Both of you need to eliminate the tendency to see feedback as failure or judgment. It is all just *feedback* so that you can both experience the most incredible pleasure possible, states Bratton.

Women often require sensual, passionate, and unrushed sex in order to climax. Move slowly, stimulate her nipples, look her in the eyes and connect with her emotionally. Do not pound against her -- harder and faster do not equate to better for a woman. Neither does "going deep"-- the inner two thirds of the vagina are substantially less sensitive than the outer third. Reassure her often during core-play, foreplay, and sex by telling her how gorgeous she is and how much she turns you on. If she gives you oral sex, do not take that as permission to climax! Think of it as a light snack before the actual act.

Above all else, never forget the importance of stimulating her clitoris throughout intercourse. All her pleasure nerves are attached to her clitoris, and dozens of studies have demonstrated that women who receive direct clitoral stimulation during intercourse are far more likely to climax consistently. Experiment with positions that will grind your body up against her clitoris (strategically placed pillows can help here), manually stimulate her when entering her from behind, use a vibrator at times, and encourage her to pleasure herself should she desire to do so. Some women are self-conscious about this, so let her know it turns you on when she touches herself. Finally, after the final act, don't turn over and immediately pass out. Tell her you love her, and cuddle with her for at least a few minutes.

Following the advice in this chapter will vastly increase your woman's chances of having multiple orgasms and of climaxing during intercourse. If your woman has never been able to climax in the past, it may not happen immediately for her. However, if you continue to follow these guidelines she will learn to relax and let go, and the constant feedback she provides you will allow you to master her body so that she can come with ease every time. Never put pressure on her to climax though, and keep in mind her body was not built for easy orgasms from penetration like yours was.

I believe the following excerpt from Ian Kerner's book *She Comes First* sums up the guidelines in this chapter perfectly:

Cunnilinguist Manifesto

A call to action that urges us first and foremost to:
- *Respect the female process of arousal*
- *Postpone gratification in the pursuit of mutual pleasure*
- *Know and appreciate the clitoris in all its manifold aspects*
- *Stimulate the clitoris appropriately through the entire process of sexual response*

- *Dispense with the conventional wisdom that exalts genital penetration as the apogee of sexual pleasure*
- *Purge yourself of stereotypes, clichés, and prejudices*
- *Be patient, respectful, sensitive and tender*
- *Take an approach that is pleasure-oriented, not goal-oriented*
- *Approach each act as a unique process of giving and receiving, knowing and learning*
- *Give of yourself seriously, generously, and wholeheartedly, even if your relationship is casual and impermanent*

If you follow this guide, you will be rewarded with an extremely sexually-satisfied woman, a stronger bond, a happier relationship, and greater sexual frequency. You may never hear her say "I'm not in the mood" again!

Chapter 13
Maximizing His Pleasure

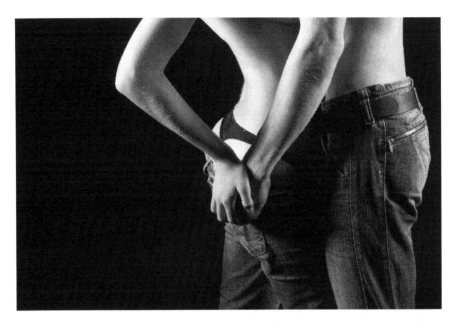

Although 95% of men report climaxing during sexual encounters, 41% still claim they are sexually dissatisfied. Even if your man is part of the "satisfied" group, it doesn't mean you can't enhance his pleasure even further!

Just Say Yes

One of the biggest sexual complaints that men in relationships have is lack of frequency. As mentioned earlier in the book, having sex will help to reactivate your libido and lead to the desire for more sex. If you're in a rut, and have been rejecting your man more often than not lately, just say yes. Don't do it as a "favor" though, do it for your mutual pleasure. Insist on oral sex first, make sure he brings you to climax before entering you, and initiate positions during intercourse that rub your clitoris and feel the best for you (knowing that you're into it will maximize his pleasure as well). Have him study and follow the guidelines in Chapter 10 and prepare yourself for the best sex of your life!

Communicate

Surveys show pleasing you is his biggest sexual desire, and the easiest, most effective way to allow him to do so is with open communication. Talk to him outside the bedroom and let him know that your needs change constantly, and you want to provide him feedback during sex so that you can both experience the most incredible pleasure possible. Tell him not to take any feedback as failure or judgment; it is simply guidance, so he can adapt to your fluctuating needs.

Teach Him What You Want

Insecurity is every bit as common in men as it is in women and understanding how to please you sexually is one of the biggest ego boosters possible. Men like it when you are direct, so don't be afraid to speak up during foreplay and sex and tell him exactly what you want him to do. And when he does something that turns you on or feels good, let him know, either with words or moans of pleasure. Also, don't be afraid of telling him if something he is doing isn't working for you. If he is sensitive and you are worried about offending him, try saying something like "baby do this instead" or "I like this ___ better." You can also grab his hand and show him where and how to place it, guide his hips while inside of you, and initiate sex position changes.

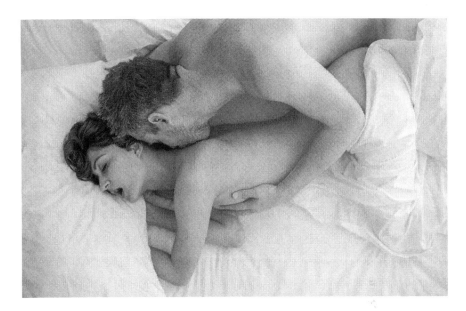

Talk Dirty

Most men love it when their partners moan, groan and talk dirty to them. Silence can make a man feel like he is not pleasing you, and as mentioned above, the number one goal of most men is to please his woman. When it comes to dirty talk, it does not need to be vulgar; what you say is not as important as how you say it.

You can build tension outside the bedroom and have him thinking about you all day long by whispering in a sultry, sexy voice "I want you so badly right now," or "I can't wait to get you inside of me," or "I can't wait to blow your mind tonight." During foreplay and sex, simply affirming your pleasure by saying "Yes baby, that's amazing" or "More" or "Just like that" with a sultry tone will dramatically increase his arousal. If your tendency is to be quiet in bed, this may feel awkward at first, but with time you will become more comfortable with it and will likely find it enhances your pleasure as well.

Initiate Sex

Studies show men initiate sex twice as often as women. They also show the more frequently either partner initiates sex, the more pleased they both tend to be with each other. Men like to feel desirable and attractive too, and when you initiate sex it can be a real ego boost for him. Initiating sex has also been found to be a libido booster for the initiator, so it's a win-win situation. What are you waiting for? Go grab your man!

Allow Him to Watch You

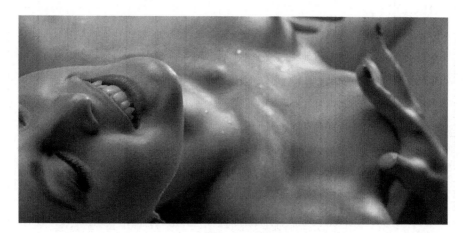

Arousal for men is largely visually based, and watching you please yourself is a huge turn on for most men. It is also one of the best ways for him to learn what pleases you. Instruct him to pay attention to how you please and stroke yourself and to note how hard, how fast, what fingers or parts of the hands are used, and what rhythms and motions bring you to orgasm.

Tease Him and Explore His Entire Body

Men are always being told to explore the entire female body, and the same rule applies here for women. Play with and suck on his nipples; explore his chest and abdomen; blow, lick and nibble his ears and neck; spend some time kissing and caressing his hip bones, lower abdomen and inner thighs; and don't forget his testicles. Teasing him for a while with kisses, licks and caresses everywhere accept for his genital area will help to create extraordinary sexual tension, and ecstasy when you finally do give him oral sex.

Give Him Ecstasy-Inducing Oral Sex

Fellatio is the easiest way for a woman to stimulate a man to orgasm, and numerous surveys show men enjoy fellatio as much as, if not more than, intercourse. Your man may be tempted to orgasm during oral sex but let him know he is not allowed to do so. Talk to him outside the bedroom and tell him you are giving him oral for both of your pleasure, but it is meant to be foreplay and followed up with cunnilingus and/or intercourse, otherwise you will be left unsatisfied. Tell him if he feels himself getting close, it is his job to stop you and to initiate other sexual activities. For an extra treat you may want to occasionally surprise him with a fellatio session where you allow him to climax, and on those occasions, you should let him know by telling him you want him to come for you. Now let's explore the techniques for giving him the best oral sex of his life.

One of the most important things you can do is to stop thinking of blow jobs as a job. If he senses that you are not enjoying yourself it is a major pleasure inhibitor for him, and most men report enthusiasm as the number one quality of an incredible blow job. Focus on how wonderful it is to provide him with such ecstatic pleasure and let yourself get turned on in the process.

Before giving him oral, tease him briefly by licking him over his underwear or licking in between his legs where his thigh meets his groin. Kiss all around his penis, then just when he thinks you are about to give him oral sex, move back up to his lips for a brief moment. Don't do this for too long though, because excessive teasing can be frustrating for a man. That doesn't mean you shouldn't build tension and anticipation by exploring his entire body; it simply means once you make your way to his groin area, men generally prefer you get down to business.

Occasionally look up at him during fellatio and give an erotic and affirmative glance. Avoid using your teeth at all costs and use your saliva to make it as wet as possible. Use your hands during oral to gently play with his testicles or to stimulate the shaft of his penis. The head is the most sensitive part, so be gentle with it. The shaft is the least sensitive part, so you can gradually apply more pressure to it. Use a variety of licks, sucks, rhythms and pressure levels (soft, hard, wet, fast, intermittent etc.), and alternate between stimulating just the shaft or just the head, to stimulating the entire penis with your mouth and dominant hand.

All men are different, so pay close attention to his responses (moaning, breathing, tightening of the abdomen, moving his body towards or away from you etc.) and adapt your techniques accordingly. Communicate with him as well, ask him for feedback in the moment, and ask him to tell you what he likes.

For more tips and techniques for pleasing your man check-out Personallifemedia.com.

And for oral sex specific tips see: https://personallifemedia.com/2017/02/60-tantalizing-bj-techniques.

Chapter 14
Sex Toys, Fantasies and Other Ways to Spice Up Your Love Life

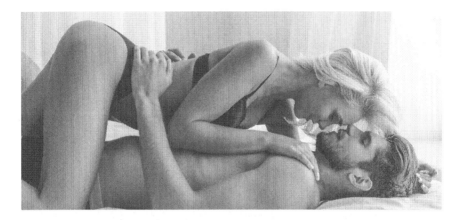

Maximizing mutual pleasure starts with open and honest communication and an establishment of desires and boundaries. Increased healthy sexual activity requires a clear request for love making, and always remember -- no means no. Now let's have some fun!

Use Lubrication

Lubrication is extremely important for a woman's comfort and pleasure, and if she is not naturally very lubricated or you engage in intercourse for an extended period of time, you should have lube on hand. Virgin coconut oil is my favorite all-natural lubricant. K-Y jelly is one of the most common store-bought lubricants, but I don't recommend it because it can dry out too quickly. Astroglide® is better because it provides lasting protection from friction during long lovemaking sessions.

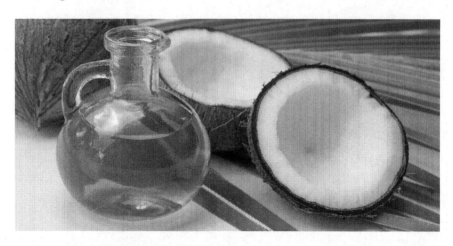

Don't Be Afraid to Fantasize

Some people feel guilty about fantasizing during sex (especially if that fantasy involves another lover), but it is completely natural and healthy, and can enhance the sexual experience. In fact, studies have found that approximately 85% of men and women have sexual fantasies during intercourse at least some of the time.[114] They have also found that people who fantasize during sex experience greater sexual satisfaction and fewer sexual problems in their relationship.

Role Play

Role playing is a fun way to keep things fresh and new and add some excitement into your love life. Ask your partner about her fantasies and openly share yours. Some fun ones to consider include doctor/patient, nurse/patient,

---

[114] http://www.tandfonline.com/doi/abs/10.1080/00224490109552069

professor/student, pirate/captor, client/call girl, the repairman, fireman, porn stars, dominant/submissive, and strangers at a bar.

Get a Little Rough

Occasionally getting a little rough can be a huge turn-on for both men and women when in a loving and committed relationship. Men, you may want to experiment with gently pulling her hair, spanking her, pushing her up against a wall, and ripping her clothes off. Women, don't be afraid to experiment with getting frisky as well. Try pulling his hair, using his body for your pleasure only, gently nibbling his neck, lips or nipples, and/or tearing off his clothes. In the context of a loving relationship, these acts can make your partner feel extremely irresistible (like you just can't control yourself because you are too overwhelmed with desire), and that can be a huge ego boost. Make sure to pay very close attention to your partner's reactions though, because not everyone enjoys this type of behavior.

Use Sex Toys

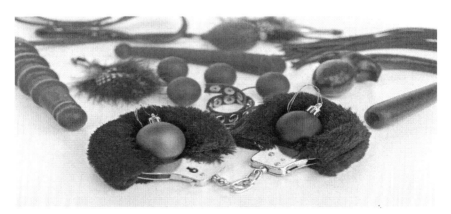

Men need to get over their fear of sex toys and the idea that they will be replaced by them. There are things that a sex toy can do that a man simply can't and using them will help ensure both partners have mind blowing orgasms. If you are new to the world of sex toys, I recommend you start off with a vibrator, such as the Hitachi Magic Wand, which can be used during cunnilingus and also during intercourse. Contact our office as we can get you the best make of vibrator that most women prefer.

Another great one for female pleasure are rings that you slip around the base of a man's penis that have a vibrator built right into them. With the proper positioning during sex, this can provide excellent clitoral stimulation. Also try using a sex toy designed specifically for the stimulation of the G-spot. Butt plugs are another fun experimental toy to try. And if you want to be really adventurous, the women can strap on a dildo and give the man anal penetration. This is a great way to change up the power in the bedroom and to experience something new.

Use a BlindFold

Blindfolds can help you really tune into the sensations you are experiencing in your body and they give you a chance to let go of control and allow your partner to take over. Take turns with the blindfold, and if you are the one who is blindfolded, try lying back and just enjoying the experience of not knowing what your partner will do next. If you are the one without the blindfold, tease your partner by touching and kissing her or his entire body before you give them oral sex or enter them.

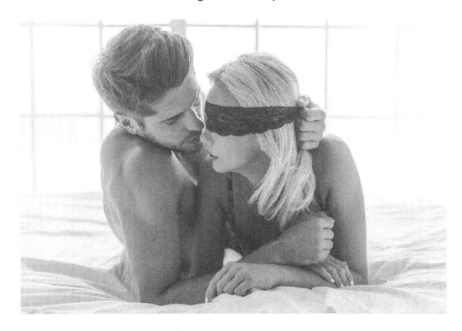

Engage in Mutual Masturbation

Watching each other masturbate is not only a huge turn-on for most couples, as mentioned above, it is also one of the best ways to learn what pleases your partner. Pay attention to where and how your partner touches him or herself. Notice how it changes as he or she comes closer to climaxing and incorporate these techniques when making love to your partner.

Play Teacher/Student

A great way to enhance your sexual chemistry is to teach each other what you like. Take turns playing the teacher and student, with the teacher dictating where and how to touch, what positions to use, how to give oral sex, and how to move during intercourse. When you are the student, have your partner guide your hands and lips to his or her preferred pleasure zones and allow your partner to dictate the rhythm and motion of oral sex and penetration.

Participate in Affectionate, Non-Sexual Touch

Babies who are not touched and held fail to thrive, and the requirement for touch and affection continues throughout life. Touch helps to relax you and your partner, it creates a sense of wellbeing, and it bonds and connects you in a way that no conversation can. Hold hands, kiss often, caress each other's hair, hug, and cuddle, whenever you get the chance!

Do Something Outdoors in the Sunlight

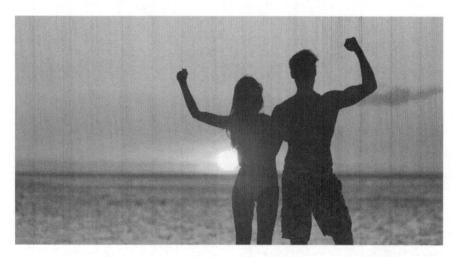

This suggestion may sound strange, but it is important because not only does sunlight improve your mood, it also increases LH hormone which stimulates the release of testosterone According to one study, sunlight exposure alone may triple sexual satisfaction.[115]

Learn and Cater to Her Love Language

This one may not sound sexy, but believe me, learning how to communicate love to your partner will translate positively into the bedroom and likely lead to more frequent and pleasurable sex. According to Gary Chapman, there are five languages of love: words of affirmation, acts of service, receiving gifts, quality time, and physical touch.

A person's love language is the way in which they receive and communicate their love. Your love language is likely different than your partner's, and if you don't understand and cater to your partner's language, it can create a lot of misunderstandings and unnecessary difficulties. For instance, let's say your love language is "acts of service" and your partner's is "words of affirmation." You may have spent the entire day "proclaiming" your love to your partner by cooking dinner and tidying the house, but your partner may still feel unloved because you haven't verbally told them how much you love them. If you try to initiate sex when your partner is feeling neglected, their instinct will be to pull away, or to engage but not wholeheartedly.

Once you understand your partner's love language, making him or her feel loved will become super easy and straightforward, you will argue way less frequently, and your love life will benefit as a result. You can discover your love language for free and get a copy of the best-selling book here: http://www.5lovelanguages.com/

Have Sex Outside the Bedroom

Keep things exciting and interesting by having sex in new places. For more inhibited couples this could simply mean having sex in the shower, on the kitchen counter, up against a wall, in front of a mirror. . . or one of my personal favorites -- on top of an operating washing machine. For the more adventurous types, perhaps you could try having sex in the ocean or lake, in the woods, at a park (when no one is around of course), or at your parents' house (the oh-so-wrong feeling, can feel oh-so-right!).

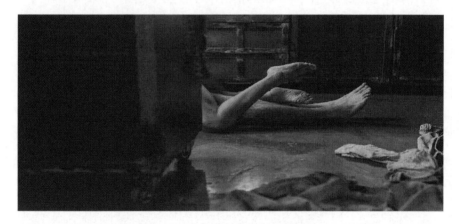

Take Amore-V

Amore V is a powerful, safe and all-natural supplement that will allow for mutually mind-blowing sex that lasts all night. It contains a special blend of concentrated herbs that clear enzymes which interfere with nitric oxide, which as discussed earlier, is a neurotransmitter that plays a major role in arousal, pleasure and sexual function. This product allows both partners to engage in sex for extended periods of time and will reduce the refractory period between erections and orgasms, enhance vaginal lubrication, and increase clitoral and penile pleasure sensations. Men and women report a fuller romantic experience upon taking the capsule one hour prior to intimate stimulation. *see appendix for ordering info

Ditch the Missionary Position

The missionary position is one of the most common sex positions, and yet it is the absolute worst for female pleasure because it doesn't allow for stimulation of the clitoris. The ideal sex positions for mutually pleasurable sex either leave space for manual stimulation of the clitoris or allows the clitoris to rub against the man's body.

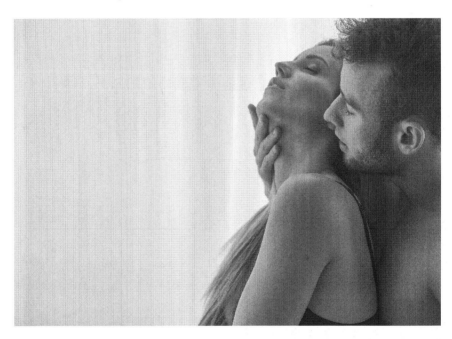

Try Different Positions

Avoid falling into a rut where you repeat the same 'go-to' positions nearly every time. Try some new and crazy positions such as the wheelbarrow or X-factor (a quick google search will reveal thousands of additional positions to play with). Find ones that please you both and tweak them to make them your own.

Videotape Yourselves

Having a video camera setup to capture you in the act can bring a whole new level of excitement to the bedroom. It is also fun to watch afterwards, and may just lead to rounds 2, 3, and 4! Be sure you inform your partner and your partner agrees to be on private camera.

For free access to exclusive interviews with doctors and expert practitioners on love, intimacy, sexual techniques, hormones, herbs and supplements that enhance the sexual experience, TUNE IN TO: https://www.youtube.com/user/DelgadoVideo/search?query=sex

Part 4
Enhancing Emotional, Physical and Spiritual Intimacy

Chapter 15
Enhancing Intimacy & Mutual Bliss
with Kundalini

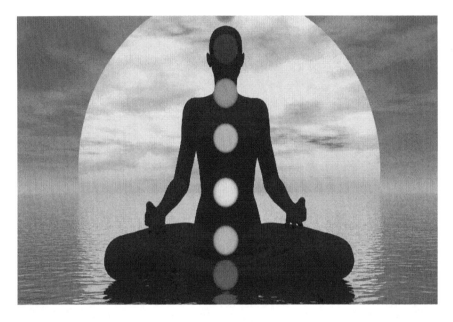

Sexual energy is life force energy. It is considered by many cultures to be the ultimate healing energy and the most powerful force available to man. Sex is a doorway for the awakening of this energy and learning how to use sex to do so will provide you and your partner with impalpable ecstasy and with a profound sense of intimacy and unity.

Sexual energy is not simply about the sexual act though. It determines how you engage with life, how you create, how you connect, how expressive you are, how open you are, and how you give and experience love. It also determines how attractive you are. It is that certain "Je ne sais quoi" that some people have that makes them irresistible, regardless of their physical appearance. It is transformative, fertile, and forever changing.

Stagnant Sexual Energy

Most people have negative emotions and perceptions embedded in their minds, which prevents the flow of sexual energy. When sexual energy is blocked or stagnant, the vibration and the frequency in your body slows down. This causes you to experience great disharmony in your life and in your relationships.

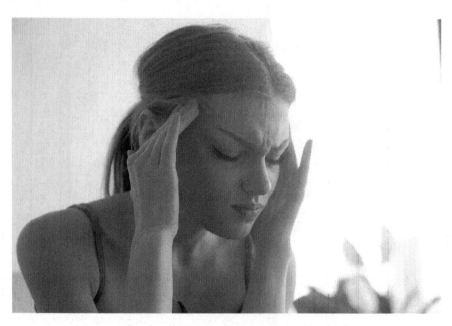

Stagnant sexual energy can manifest as sexual dysfunction and lead to a loss of desire or arousal, or an inability to perform or to orgasm. It can also manifest as an inability to commit, an inability to fully give or receive love, defensiveness, manipulation, resistance, emotional walls, a lack of creativity, insecurity, addiction, disease, and great difficulty in achieving one's dreams and goals.

Kundalini and Tantric Sex: The Basics

Most people have heard of Kundalini and tantric sex, but few people fully understand what it is. Kundalini refers to a primal, sexual energy that is located at the base of the spine. Awakening this energy is said to lead to enlightenment. Tantra refers to ancient customs and practices of Hinduism. Tantric sex is a form of ritualized sacred sex that stems from Hinduism, and its practice can awaken the Kundalini energy.

Tantra teaches you how to harness and cultivate your sexual energy to its deepest potential which transcends pleasure and procreation. It emphasizes awareness and the importance of the present moment. Refilling your body with deep sexual energy allows you to experience your core essence, to see that you are directly connected to everything, and to experience another as yourself. When you heighten your sexual energy, harmony is restored and everything in your life falls into place. Your heart's desires become achievable, and you are able to experience a whole-hearted connection with your lover and mutual ecstasy.

Below is a summary of some of the fundamental teachings of Kundalini and tantric sex, in no particular order. You can use these teachings to cultivate your own sexual energy and to formulate a deep level of connectivity and intimacy with your partner. Please keep in mind however, that this is just a brief outline of a few teachings. To truly understand Kundalini and all its wisdoms would take a lifetime of study and practice.

Teaching 1 – Emphasize the Journey

Modern sex is typically based exclusively on satisfying physical urges. It is done without consciousness. Because there is often a disconnect between partners, it provides a mere fraction of the pleasure that Kundalini-awakened sex (which incorporates the mind, body and soul) can provide. Although practicing tantric sex will most certainly enhance your own pleasure, it should not be practiced with the intent of doing so. The fundamental idea of Kundalini is that sex should be a selfless act of love, enjoyed slowly, without expectations or goals. When practicing tantric sex, it is the journey, not the destination that counts.

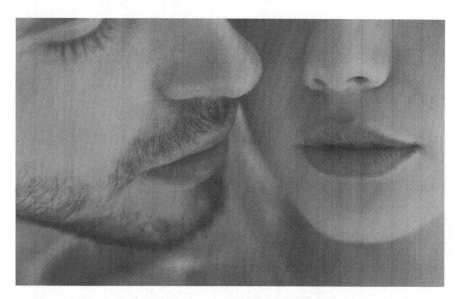

Teaching 2 - Shift the Focus from Orgasms

Most of us are addicted to orgasms. We want more, we want better, we want faster. We use orgasms not just for pleasure, but also to temporarily forget our problems, and to relieve stress and anxiety. According to spiritual counselor, awakened sexuality mentor, and conscious relationship guide Zeerak Khan, there is a deeper, underlying reason why we are so addicted to orgasms though: that reason is that orgasms force your mind to stop and place you in the present moment.

During orgasms your personality momentarily forgets itself. You briefly enter a space of oneness where your heart is fully open, and you are fully connected to your lover and to the universe. In that place of presence and oneness, your ego (which is the chief source of human suffering), is temporarily dissolved. All of your perceived problems and all of the things you feel are lacking in your life disappear. Love, pleasure, and fulfillment is all that exists.

At this point you're probably thinking that what I just said about orgasms is fantastic, but there are a few major drawbacks. Firstly, sexual energy is the most powerful and potent source of vital life force energy, and orgasms deplete that force. A hyper-focus on orgasms is also problematic because it is only about yourself, and the natural tendency is to disconnect immediately after orgasming.

Chasing orgasms prevents you from being in the moment, having a depth of connection, and creating true intimacy with your partner. While foregoing orgasms is not a practical recommendation for most, you can help preserve and cultivate your sexual energy by delaying your orgasms and by shifting your focus. Instead of orgasm-oriented sex, place all your focus and awareness on being fully in the moment with your lover.

Teaching 3 - Take It Slow

Men are fueled by testosterone, and one of testosterone's main functions is to increase reaction time (which was necessary in the past to react quickly in danger). This primal need to speed things up often translates into the bedroom, where foreplay is rushed or skipped, and intercourse is hard and fast. Unfortunately, this type of sexual behavior is reinforced by pornography, where more often than not, foreplay is skipped or includes only oral sex given by the woman to the man, followed by rough and fast intercourse. The women in these films are often screaming with pleasure, but these women are actors being paid to pretend.

Women's bodies don't work that way; women need to be showered with attention, affection and loving touch in order to release the oxytocin that is required to relax their bodies and ready them for sex. The longer you spend in the foreplay stage, the more energy you will build together and within, and the end result is greater pleasure for both of you. Intercourse should also be slower, and softer, and as mentioned above the ultimate goal should not be orgasm -- any type of goal orientation will leave you feeling depleted. Instead, focus on the intimacy, connection and pleasure-sharing that is occurring in the moment between you two.

Teaching 4 - Be in the Moment

Tantric sex is all about presence and awareness. Before even beginning foreplay, both partners should take a few moments to breath and relax. Imagine yourself breathing in positivity and breathing out lingering stressors of the day. Bring your awareness to your heart, focus on love, and try to feel your heart opening. If you find it hard to stay in the moment, shift from thinking to feeling. Ask yourself: "How does it feel to be in this body?" And then feel the pleasure your body is providing you. Ask yourself: "How does it feel to be in this experience?" And then feel that pleasure as well, recommends Khan. At the same time, know that you are not your feelings, sensations or thoughts. You are a spiritual being experiencing your true self through your body.

Stare into your partner's eyes and feel the depths of love build between you. Let go of all the thoughts that bombard your brain. When you find your mind wandering, simply refocus your attention on your partner, on the magic of the moment, and on the bond between you two. Whatever comes up, whatever arises, just allow it to be in the periphery. When you learn to be fully present in the moment, you will experience your true self and the incredible depths of pleasure and ecstasy will become available to you.

Teaching 5 - Practice Eye Gazing and Deep Breathing

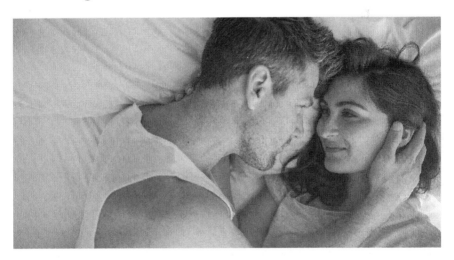

Extended eye contact is an essential part of tantric sex and deep connection in intimacy. It brings you into the moment and allows you to see beyond the physical, into your partner's soul. It also forces you to let your guard down, to be vulnerable, and to let your partner see you wholly. During foreplay, hold eye contact for two to five minutes and resist the temptation to look away. And during intercourse try to engage in extended eye contact as often as possible.

According to Wendy Strgar, in her book *Love that Works: A Guide to Enduring Intimacy,* "It is surprisingly harder to do than you might expect. Move toward this idea as an intention rather than a rule and be amazed as the collection of glimpses that will reshape how you think about your partner and yourself. It is not easy to be seen, even by the people we love.Truly witnessing the act of love is profoundly transformative."

Another important step for connecting and building sexual energy is breathing deeply. Babies breathe right down to their bellies, but most children and adults breathe using only their chests. This lifelong distorted breathing depletes the lifeforce and creates an energetic shutdown. Reconnecting to the breath and breathing not only deeply but also in harmony with your partner will build your life force and keep you connected and in the moment. For harmonized breathing, all you have to do is bring your mouths close together and inhale while your partner exhales. Allow his or her breath to travel down your entire body, and consciously energize and share your breath in return.

Teaching 6 - Worship and Explore the Entire Body

With tantra, intercourse is downplayed, and foreplay becomes coreplay. The longer you spend in the foreplay stage, the more energy you will build together and within, and the end result is greater pleasure for both of you. Spend extended amounts of time exploring each other's entire body, while avoiding the typical 'erogenous' zones. Caress each other's feet and hands, feel all the fingers and both palms, and tune into the feeling of the nerve endings at the tips of your fingers. Tell your partner what feels good, linger in your partner's touch, and let yourself be completely vulnerable and open to your partner.

With time, you may slowly progress to the erogenous zones, but remember the goal is not orgasm. Instead, focus on the intimacy, connection and pleasure-sharing that is occurring in the moment between you two. Make intercourse slower and softer, and delay orgasm as long as possible. If you feel yourself getting close, use your breath to relax, reconnect to your partner, and recenter yourself.

Teaching 7- Surrender Yourself Wholly

In order to activate the Kundalini energy and experience mutual ecstasy, you need to yield, surrender, and open yourself up completely to your partner. During foreplay and sex, focus on the sensations in your physical, emotional, and spiritual body. Allow yourself to really experience the deep level of acceptance, passion and love that is occurring and the acknowledgment of knowing that you and your partner are one (not separate from each other). Relax your body and your mind, fall into the moment, and accept whatever happens next. If you are the type of person who feels uncomfortable receiving pleasure or worries that you are being self-indulgent at the expense of your partner, don't. Love is a state of unity, and because your partner loves you, giving you pleasure provides them with pleasure.

Teaching 8 - Dispel Shame and Embrace Your Sexuality

According to Khan, sex has been separated from its core essence which is spirituality. Organized religions are a major cause of this separation. Many religions preach that sex is just meant for procreation, sexuality is sinful, and to be closer to God you must suppress your sexuality. Marketing and the media further separate sex from spirituality by exploiting it for money. This leads to a negative duality where we're either stifling sex or selling it, says Khan. As a result, there are many negative connotations associated with sex and sexuality, a few of which include shame, fear, and guilt.

These connotations cause many of us to suppress our sexuality. And the more we suppress and repress it, the more we are in our guilt, the more we are in our shame, the more it comes out in destructive ways, says Khan. We must remember the core of our being started with sexuality. And sexual energy is an extremely powerful, positive, healing energy. It is highly creative energy, and reconnecting to your sexuality shows you the true nature of who you really are, which is love. Let go of fear, shame, and guilt. Admire your naked body, and fully embrace your experience as a sensual and sexual being.

Teaching 9 - Understand That Resistance is Natural

When you truly love someone and allow yourself to become one with them, mind, body and soul, a lot of resistance will surface. Love has an effect of reconnecting you to your spirit, and when you bring the spirit through with love, it brings up everything inside of you that you have not yet resolved and is challenging your ability to love. All kinds of past pains and negative experiences that you buried deep in your subconscious mind will come to the surface, and those negative feelings are often (misappropriately) directed towards your partner.

This is why challenges so often arise the moment a couple starts to have sex - the level of intimacy that occurs during sex accelerates the surfacing of repressed emotions and experiences. Knowing that the negative feelings are not caused by your partner is essential for a lasting, happy relationship. If you notice a lot of negativity, nitpicking, or agitation towards your partner, remind yourself that your partner is a reflection of you and you are likely projecting onto your partner. The quickest way to overcome these unconscious responses is by reprogramming your subconscious mind with tools such as hypnosis, positive affirmations, and our LFC eyes open hypnosis scripts.

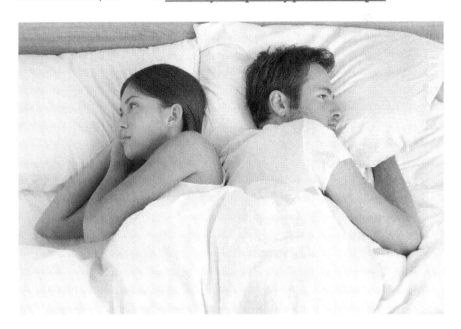

Teaching 10 - - Embrace the Healing Nature of Sexual Energy

Sexual energy is not only the most powerful force we have, it is also highly therapeutic. When used consciously, it can be a great catalyst for spiritual growth, healing, and transformation on all levels. To engage in conscious, healing sex, you need to yield, surrender, and open yourself up completely to your partner. Use harmonizing breaths and eye gazing to deepen your connection. Allow your partner to take over your whole body and trust that his or her main motivation is to show you love and give you pleasure.

The healing nature of conscious sex may trigger deep emotions such as sadness, fear, anger or pain. These emotions are stuck energetically in the body, and when they arise, you are accessing and healing your pain body. This may cause you to cry, and you should let yourself do so. Embracing all of your feelings allows you to process and release them. It clears out negative, old energy, reawakens and opens your heart, and paves the way to true connectivity and ecstasy.

Teaching 11 - Recognize the Ego

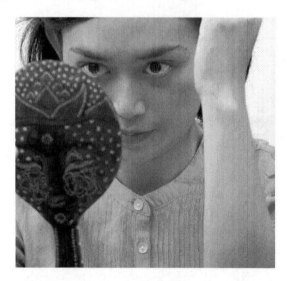

The ego causes you to identify yourself as an isolated being, incomplete and separate from self and others. It prevents you from seeing your true nature, as a whole and complete being. The ego is based externally and seeks to find happiness from outside sources, instead of finding it from within. The separation that the ego causes leads to jealousy, fear, and drama in relationships. It also causes tremendous suffering and prevents you from experiencing true happiness and peace.

Because the insecure and fragile ego is survival-based, it can cause you to guard your heart and hold back parts of yourself as a protective mechanism. But never fully letting someone in prevents you from formulating deep, whole-hearted love connections. An important part of tantra is recognizing the role the ego plays in your emotions and behaviors and learning to disregard the ego's beliefs and urges.

* For my VIP clients I create a personalized script using Time Line Therapy and NLP to release negative emotions and replace them with powerful loving emotions. It works incredibly well for resolving guilt, anger, hurt etc.

Teaching 12 - Let Go of Fear and Manipulation

Sadness, rejection, failure, and heartache are a natural and unavoidable part of the human experience. Unfortunately, when you experience them, it causes a part of yourself to shut down, and you become overtaken by fear. Fear that you are not loveable, fear that you will lose your partner, and fear that you are lacking in love. Operating from a place of fear depletes your life force energy and prevents you from seeing that you are already loved, whole and complete.

Your ego responds to fear defensively, and this causes you to manipulate and control your partner and other loved ones in attempt to keep your love sources around. Your ego may also respond by withholding love or by using sexuality to temporarily gratify and feel connected. In order to cultivate sexual energy and formulate a deep, loving relationship, you need to dispel fear and the compulsion to control and manipulate.

Teaching 13 – Take Responsibility for Your Pain

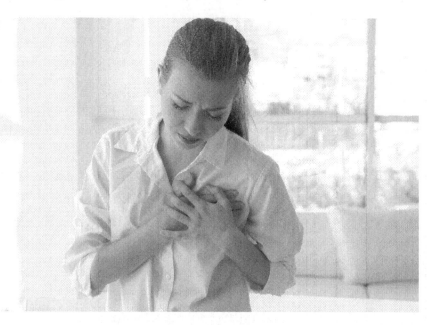

You are responsible for your feelings, and no one can "make" you feel anything. Your ego doesn't understand this though, and it prefers to project your pain onto your partner. You blame him or her for your negative feelings, and you look to your partner to make you feel happy and whole – which is impossible. You need to recognize that pain is your responsibility and understand that your partner didn't elicit that pain. Don't try to suppress pain; it is a natural part of the human experience. Instead, when pain arises, observe it, embrace it, be with it, and know that in a few moments or a few days, it will transmute and disappear.

Teaching 14 - Recognize That We Are One

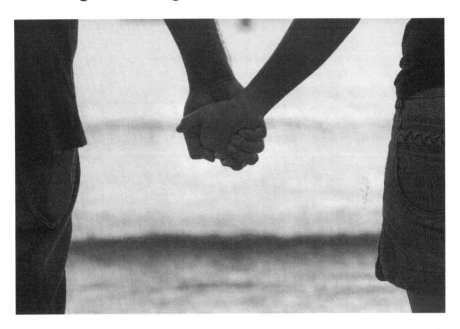

Ego creates separation, and it is the primary source of human pain, fear, and suffering. Incorporating the teachings of Kundalini into your life will allow you to dissolve your ego, to see that you are a part of a whole, and that we are all connected as one. It will allow you to see into your partner and to see beyond your partner. Where your partner ends and where you begin will dissolve. And you'll realize that whatever you do to your partner, you are essentially doing to yourself. Because you will no longer experience your partner as separate, you will no longer feel the need to control them or change them, and you will stop projecting onto them. You will release feelings of jealousy, fear, and distrust, and you will allow them to be exactly as they are.

Whenever you feel ego-driven emotions and compulsions arising, refer to the teachings of Kundalini, and remind yourself you are one with the universe, you are whole, you are perfect, and you are loved.

Chapter 16
The Relationship and Health Benefits of Self-Pleasuring

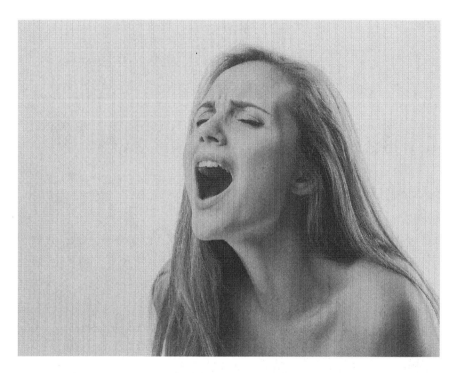

Many of us were taught growing up that masturbation is something that is dirty or wrong, or that it's something that should be done in secret and never talked about. And sadly, for women, there is an even stronger stigma attached to masturbation which leaves many feeling guilty or shameful about it. This is unfortunate because the health and relationship benefits for both genders are numerous, and masturbation itself is completely natural. In fact, touching your genitals for pleasure is something that you start doing before you even leave the womb.[116] And surveys show the vast majority of adults (94% of men and 85% of women) participate in it. It is time we let go of the negative connotations, anxiety, and discomfort we attach to masturbation and embrace it for the relationship enhancing, pleasurable, health elixir that it is.

Physical Health Benefits

Masturbation helps to lower blood pressure, relieve insomnia, reduce menstrual cramps, and improve immune system function by stimulating cortisol release.[117] [118] It relieves pain by increasing endorphin output, and recent research suggests it may even lower type-2 diabetes risk.[119] [120]

The orgasms masturbation produces increases pelvic floor strength and blood circulation to the genitals – both of which improve pleasure and orgasmic intensity. It also helps tighten the vaginal muscles in women, making sex more pleasurable for both partners. Masturbation is particularly beneficial for men who struggle with premature ejaculation. It can be used to learn the "start-stop technique" which teaches men how to control their orgasms, or if engaged in a few hours before sex, to delay orgasms during intercourse.

---

[116] https://www.smh.com.au/lifestyle/life-and-relationships/m06aboutlastnight-20170421-gvpkp9.html
[117] https://www.diabetes.co.uk/news/2013/Dec/masturbation-could-lower-diabetes-risk-91791016.html
[118] https://www.psychologytoday.com/ca/blog/stress-and-sex/201401/touchy-subject-the-health-benefits-masturbation
[119] https://www.diabetes.co.uk/news/2013/Dec/masturbation-could-lower-diabetes-risk-91791016.html
[120] http://theconversation.com/happy-news-masturbation-actually-has-health-benefits-16539

Masturbation also helps reduce the risk for cervical and urinary tract infections in women because the opening of the cervix and contractions that occur during orgasms help flush out bacteria-laden cervical fluids. And it reduces the risk for prostate cancer in men in a similar manner by flushing out cancer-causing toxins from the prostate gland.[121]

Mental and Emotional Benefits

Masturbation helps relieve tension and anxiety and lower stress which is a leading risk factor for most chronic diseases. It helps boost self-esteem and self-image, enhance overall well-being, and ward off depression.[122] Masturbation is able to produce such a wide-range of mental and emotional benefits because it releases numerous feel-good neurotransmitters that lift your spirits and activate the reward circuits in your brain.

An orgasm produces euphoria and a natural high, and it provides the greatest non-drug blast of dopamine available. This is beneficial because dopamine plays a key role in pleasure, motivation, libido, and happiness, and it reduces cravings for unhealthy foods and other addictive substances. Masturbation also releases oxytocin, a natural antidepressant and bliss-inducing hormone that helps you feel relaxed and loving, and builds optimism and confidence.[123] Last but not least, masturbation helps you understand your sexual needs and boundaries, which according to the European Regional

---

[121] https://www.diabetes.co.uk/news/2013/Dec/masturbation-could-lower-diabetes-risk-91791016.html

[122] https://www.psychologytoday.com/ca/blog/stress-and-sex/201401/touchy-subject-the-health-benefits-masturbation

[123] https://www.nature.com/news/neuroscience-the-hard-science-of-oxytocin-1.17813

Bureau of the WHO, enables you to communicate more clearly in sexual situations, and helps you avoid being abused.[124]

Relationship Benefits

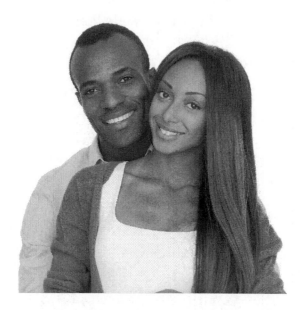

Research shows those who masturbate have more fulfilling sex lives, a better emotional and physical connection with their partners, and enhanced long-term partnerships and marriages. Masturbation helps to improve sexual response and the ability to achieve orgasm, and it's the foundation of most sex therapy. It is particularly helpful for people who have difficulty with climaxing during sex because it teaches you about your body and what feels best, and this knowledge can then be used to teach your partner how to bring you to climax.[125] A great way to teach your partner is either to

---

[124] https://www.bzga.de/infomaterialien/einzelpublikationen/?idx=2042
[125] https://www.psychologytoday.com/ca/blog/stress-and-sex/201401/touchy-subject-the-health-benefits-masturbation

masturbate in front of them or to engage in mutual masturbation and instruct them to watch you closely. You can also tell your partner verbally what to do, and/or "coach" their hand by guiding it where to go and showing it what rhythm, pace and intensity to use.

Chapter 17
Sensual Massage Techniques For Increasing Lust and Connectedness

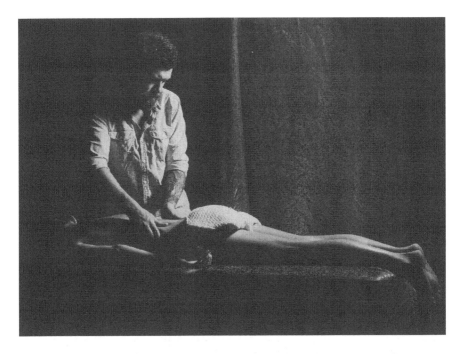

A sensual massage is one of the best ways to eliminate stress and to satisfy your partner on an emotional, physical, and spiritual level. It helps create a deeper sense of intimacy and connectivity between you two, it's a great way to dissolve any animosities leftover from an argument or fight, it fires-up the libido, and it almost always leads to amazing sex.

The Benefits

Moving into that sense of touch is so important because it activates essential hormones, the most important of which is oxytocin. In case you don't remember from Chapter 4, oxytocin plays a key role in bonding, intimacy, and attachment, and it is considered the ultimate love hormone. It is also referred to as the "cuddle hormone" because touching and cuddling is one of the best ways to release it. Oxytocin enhances relaxation and increases dopamine levels (which enhances receptivity to pleasure). It increases desire and decreases the threshold for arousal and orgasm. It also helps to make orgasms more intense and multiple orgasms easier to achieve.

If you pay close attention to your partner's responses throughout the massage (moans of pleasure etc.), you may also gain new insights into how your partner likes to be touched, and even discover unexpected erogenous zones. And men, if you're looking for a magic bullet to get your woman into the mood, this is as close as you're going to get. When you help your woman release oxytocin through a sensual massage, it releases the stresses of her day and puts her in a more free, sensual, and sexual state of mind, which means amazing sex for both of you!

Step 1: Set the Mood

Create the perfect environment by lowering the lights and using candles and/or red-light bulbs to create the optimum ambience. Make sure the temperature is ideal and eliminate any odors by opening a window for a few hours (if weather permits) or using an essential oil diffuser. Choose music that will make you both feel relaxed, yet sensual and sexy, and set the volume high enough that you can hear it but low enough that it isn't a distraction. Tidy the room and remove any potential distractions (beeping electronics etc.).

Then tend to your personal hygiene. Take a good shower because a massage enhances all the senses, and body odor will distract from your partner's ability to fully relax. Finally, turn off the phone, put some extra towels by the bed (to place underneath your partner and to wipe excess oil off your hands), and warm up some massage oil (e.g. almond oil, coconut oil, jojoba oil etc.).

Step 2: Slowly Explore Your Partner's Entire Body

A sensual massage should never be rushed and should last a bare minimum of 40 minutes. It should also include the entire body. Start with the hands, using your palm to apply long smooth strokes to the front and back of the hands. Gaze into your partner's eyes and maintain extended eye contact while doing this, to help create a sense of loving connectivity. Then work down from the tips of the fingers to the wrists, and back up to the fingers. Gently pull on each finger, and then use your thumbs to release tension in the palms.

After massaging the hands, have your partner lie on their stomach (if they aren't already doing so) and begin to massage the feet. Use your thumbs to apply pressure to all parts of the foot and gently massage and then pull on each toe. When you have finished the feet, very slowly work your way up the entire body, concentrating on one spot at a time, and include the calves, hamstrings, buttocks, lower back, upper back, wrists, arms, shoulders, neck and ears.

Step 3: Vary the Techniques

If you just use your fingers or repeat the same motion continuously, your hand muscles will get tired and your partner will get bored. Try using the palms of your hands to apply the compression technique, which simply involves pressing down on one spot to loosen the muscles in that area. You can also place one hand on top of the other and rotate in slow, circular motions. Another great technique is the stroking technique, using your entire hands in contact with your partner's body, gliding them up and down in long, gentle strokes.

If you feel knots while exploring your partner's body, place pressure on the knot using your fingers and use circular motions to help loosen them. You can also try the kneading technique to loosen knots and release tight muscles. This technique involves pressing the palms on the chosen body part, and then rolling to the base and then tips of your fingers in an upward motion, similar to kneading bread. Use different levels of pressure, friction and intensity throughout the massage; avoid any techniques that tickle or may cause pain and try to find and maintain a rhythm.

Step 4: Enter a Meditative State

Energy may not be seen by most, but it is certainly felt. Giving your partner a massage while stressed or in a negative state of mind will deter from his or her ability to fully relax. Take a few deep, relaxing breaths before even beginning the massage, and imagine your heart opening and expanding. Stay relaxed throughout the massage by breathing slowly and deeply. If you find yourself getting distracted with thoughts, try closing your eyes and tuning into your breath and her breath, breathing in tandem, as you continue the massage.

Focus on the feeling of your partner's skin, the movement of their body as they inhale and exhale, and on the pleasure of providing your partner with whole body bliss. Pay attention to any responses (sighs, moving the body towards or away from you), and adjust what you are doing accordingly. Finally, avoid being too mechanical or overthinking things -- you really can't mess up a massage that is given with love.

Step 5: Use Your Words Wisely

It is important not to talk too much during a massage -- stretches of silence help your partner become fully relaxed. That being said, well-chosen words, whispered softly, can dramatically enhance the whole experience, especially if the end goal is sex. Many women find it hard to simply sit back and let someone else give them pleasure or find it difficult to fully surrender because of body insecurities. So men if you are giving your woman a massage, put her mind at ease by telling her how much you love exploring her entire body. Tell her how beautiful her body is, how soft her skin is, how sexy her butt is, or how luscious her curves are.

If you want to make the massage extra sexy for her, whisper a sensual story in her ear in the middle of the massage. Women are turned on by auditory signals; a sensual story will stimulate many different neurotransmitters in the brain and hormones in the body which will ignite desire. If you wait until the middle of the massage to begin your story, your partner will be fully relaxed and more receptive. The story will spark her arousal, and a lusty sense of anticipation will progressively build during the rest of the massage, and by the end she will be exploding with lust and desire.

Women, you can also try whispering something sexy in your man's ear, but you don't need to share an entire story. A few simple words whispered in a sultry tone will produce impalpable sexual desire in your man, such as, "Touching you turns me on so much," or "You are so sexy," or "I love exploring your entire body," or "Your scent drives me wild." Be careful though, because just one of these statements may drive him so wild, he won't be able to enjoy the rest of the massage because he'll need to have you right away.

Chapter 18
How to Find Your Sexual and Spiritual Soulmate

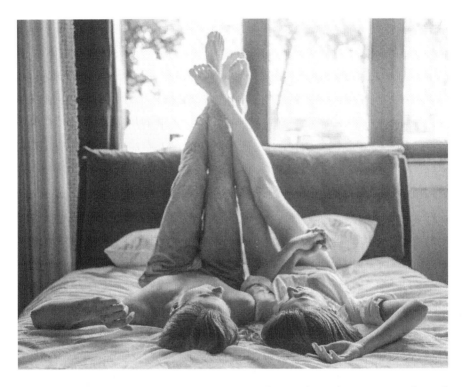

A soulmate is a person who is aligned with your soul and with whom you feel a deep energetic connection to. They help you achieve higher levels of awareness and consciousness by challenging, awakening and stirring different parts of you in a profound way. "We do our biggest learning through our relationships," explains spiritual intuitive, author and psychic to the stars Laura Powers.

Not all soulmates are sexual soulmates, but when you do find your sexual soulmate, intercourse won't just feel amazing, it will also inspire you, awaken you, and elevate you energetically. Unfortunately, no matter how desperately you want to meet your soulmate, you can't force the matter – you need to be ready. The following guidelines will help ready you for your soulmate and will create the vibrational energy that you need in order to attract your soulmate to you.

Work to Be Clear About What You Are Looking For

Many of us obsess about meeting a soulmate but fail to define what we are really looking for. Set apart a good chunk of time when you won't be disturbed to connect with your heart, and actually write down what you want in a partner. Avoid the temptation to think about what you *don't* want because whatever you focus on expands.

Think of all the positive traits you want your partner to have. You can include physical, mental, and emotional traits, and even include specifics such as what kind of job they do, what their family relationship is like, their temperament, and their passions and hobbies. Like attracts like, so be sure to refer to the list you just created and work towards achieving any traits or qualities that you are lacking.

Dive Inward

You need to align with your true self in order to draw your soulmate to you, and if your soulmate hasn't shown up, there is likely an internal block. "If you are struggling to find love and connect with it externally, you are probably struggling internally," says Laura. Instead of desperately searching for your soulmate and focusing all your energy externally, go inward. Ask yourself what it is that you are hoping your soulmate will do for you. For example, do you hope they will make you feel loveable or worthy, beautiful, complete, whole, confident, healed or secure? Whatever it is you are hoping they will do for you, recognize that these traits come from within.

Ask yourself on a scale of 1 to 100 how high would you rate your level of self-love and self-worth? If your answer is anything less than 100, than cultivating more self-love and self-worth should be your top priorities. If you don't know how to do this, try eyes-open hypnosis, time-line therapy and/or repeating certain self-affirmation scripts. They help you tap into and reprogram your subconscious mind so that you can create rapid and profound inner changes.

Love Yourself and Your Own Company

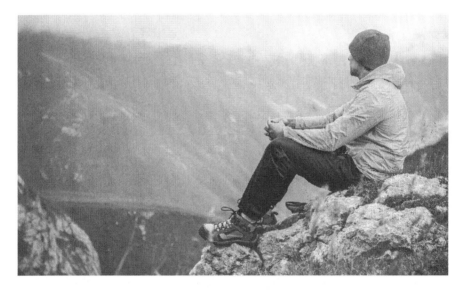

There is nothing sexier than loving yourself, enjoying your own company, and living your life to the fullest regardless of your relationship status. You need to recognize that you are beautiful, unique and amazing, and nobody is going to "add to your light" or "complete you." Try to fall in love with yourself each and every day. A great way to help with this is to start your mornings off by looking in the mirror and saying out loud "I love you, you are incredible!" . . . or something else affirming that resonates with you.

Spend time nurturing yourself, hang out with people who respect and inspire you, and do things that light you up. When you do more things that bring you joy, you will radiate with positive energy. On the other hand, if you put things off until you find a partner (like that trip to Costa Rica), and continuously worry about when or if your partner will show up, you will send out a desperate vibrational energy. This will attract unhealthy relationships and may even repel your soulmate away from you.

Learn from Your Past Relationships

Every relationship we enter into has a message or teaching for us. "We're incarnating to learn various lessons and have various experiences," states Laura. "Our largest learnings happen with immediate family and romantic partners, so we're attracting whatever it is we need to learn. So, if you're attracting a lot of patterns that are painful or there is a pattern playing out time and time again, step back and ask what is it that you need and need to learn from this." If you find yourself bouncing around from one relationship to the next, always blaming the other person for its demise, you need to recognize you are repeating unsuccessful relationship patterns because there is something you need to work on within yourself. "When you learn the lesson, that pattern will disappear."

Working through and releasing baggage from past relationships is invaluable. If you don't do this work, it can not only reduce your chances of attracting your soulmate, it can also cause you to unintentionally sabotage a soulmate relationship. Instead of villainizing your exes, take 100% responsibility. Instead of longing for or idealizing your ex, understand that it ended for a reason. Instead of holding onto a grudge, send your ex some love and be grateful for how they helped you progress on your life path. Worth noting - our significant others often act as mirrors of ourselves, so if there were things that bothered you about your ex, they are likely things you need to work on yourself.

Use the Biology of Belief

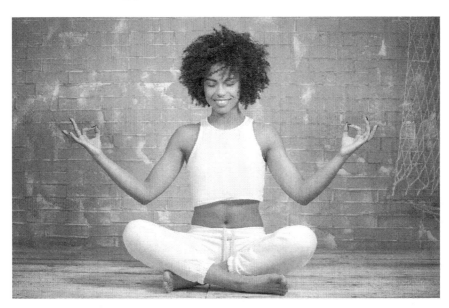

Your thoughts dictate your reality, and if you're feeding yourself negative messages such as "I'm unlovable," "I'm not good enough," "I'll never find love," or "I only attract losers," you are unconsciously blocking yourself from meeting your soulmate. Being unclear on what you want in a partner is equally problematic, because it sends mixed messages into the Universe. So, once you have taken the time to establish what you want in a partner, spend at least 20 minutes meditating on it.

If meditation is not something you regularly do, don't be scared off. All you have to do for this soulmate meditation is bring your attention to your breath and focus on breathing deeply. After about 5 to 10 minutes, or when you feel your body is fully relaxed, conjure up a picture of your soulmate. This next step is important: imagine you have already met your soulmate and see yourself with him or her. Focus on the love and joy you feel with your soulmate and feel great gratitude for having met them. Revisit the image and emotions of having found your soulmate daily, and practice the soulmate meditation weekly, and you will send a powerful signal to the Universe to bring your soulmate to you.

Release Childhood Traumas

It is nearly impossible to reach adulthood without experiencing some sort of emotional trauma and developing subconscious negative beliefs as a result. And the traumas aren't always obvious, it can be something as subtle as the feeling of being neglected once a new sibling comes along. Anything that causes emotional pain in the formative years of childhood, gets absorbed into the subconscious mind and becomes part of daily thinking and the way you view and engage with the world.

Identifying and working past childhood traumas, and reprogramming your subconscious thinking patterns towards positivity, will free you from the past and allow you to radiate a sense of inner peace. Some excellent tools to achieve this include hypnosis, a regular meditation practice, LFC hypnosis scripts (https://delgadoprotocol.com/product-store/#1523315591062-ff7ea7e6-c778), NLP, positive affirmations, and Emotional Freedom Technique.

Ditch the Birth Control Pill

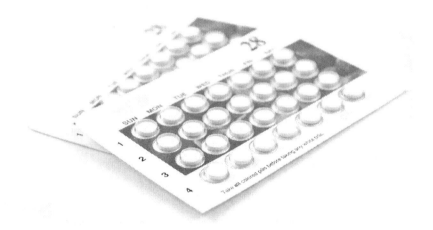

The pill may prevent you from connecting with your soulmate by skewing your subconscious ability to decipher the correct match. Major histocompatibility complex (MHC) genes, are molecules that play a role in immunity, and MHC combinations differ to varying degrees in individuals. MHC genes can be detected subconsciously in saliva when you kiss someone and also through body odor. We are subconsciously most drawn to those who have MHC combinations that are highly different from our own because dissimilar genes give offspring the best chance.[126]

The birth control pill causes the opposite effect though and shifts a woman's preference towards genetically similar

---

[126] https://www.ncbi.nlm.nih.gov/pubmed/18700206

men.[127] Unfortunately, pairing up with an MHC-similar man is associated with reduced sexual satisfaction and a higher likelihood for cheating.[128] And if you stop the pill during a relationship, the accompanying hormonal changes will drive you further away from you partner and may lead to relationship dissatisfaction or dissolution.[129] If you want a safe alternative to the birth control pill, consider using condoms, or combining the withdrawal method (don't use this on its own) with fertility awareness. There are plenty of apps available to help you with fertility awareness, but Natural Cycles is the only one that is certified for contraception.

Optimize Your Personal Biochemistry

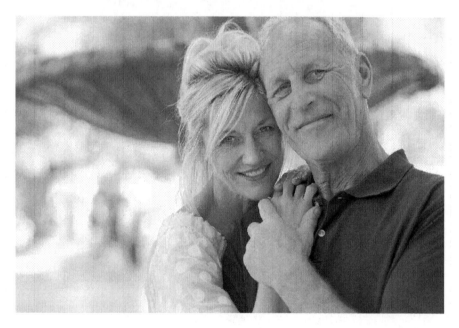

---

[127] https://www.ncbi.nlm.nih.gov/pubmed/18700206

[128] https://www.scientificamerican.com/article/birth-control-pills-affect-womens-taste/

[129] https://www.scientificamerican.com/article/birth-control-pills-affect-womens-taste/

Your soulmate is based on matters of the soul and a spiritual contract to help each other advance in your life's paths. However, as discussed earlier in the book, the euphoric feelings you get when you first fall in love with your soulmate are dictated by something much more tangible – they are dictated by chemicals in the body and brain. A cocktail of hormones and neurotransmitters plays a role in the racing heart, addictive thoughts, butterflies, giddiness, and sweaty palms.[130] If you have an imbalance of these hormones and neurotransmitters, it may hinder your ability to experience those feelings of "falling in love" and you may mistakenly reject your soulmate thinking that they can't be "the one" since they don't trigger euphoric feelings. For guidance on how to optimize your personal biochemistry refer to Chapters 5 and 6.

---

[130] https://www.sciencedaily.com/releases/2010/10/101022184957.htm

Appendix
Nutraceutical Guide for Optimizing Sexual Function, Libido and Virility

Delgado Protocol has spent decades researching, sourcing and formulating clinically proven nutraceutical supplements that effectively address the most common sexual issues. Our products are derived from the highest quality ingredients and contain no soy, no gluten, no dairy, no sugar, no GMOs, no stearates, no phosphates, no synthetic derivatives and no harmful additives. They are made using Good Manufacturing Practices (GMP), at a certified laboratory in the USA that adheres to the highest standards.

Since a high percentage of sexual dysfunction symptoms are linked to hormone imbalances, if your symptoms are ongoing and you don't yet know the cause, I recommend you take a hormone test. Hormone testing will help you to pinpoint the root cause so that you can address it with the correct nutraceutical supplement and appropriate lifestyle changes.

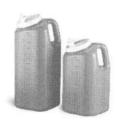

You can purchase an extremely accurate 24-hour urine kit that tests for free and total testosterone, five estrogens and all of the other key hormones that affect sexual health here: https://delgadoprotocol.com/product/24-hour-urine-analysis/.

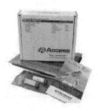

Or purchase a saliva panel test which is less costly and measures 11 key hormones here: https://delgadoprotocol.com/product/11-hormone-saliva-panel/

*The following statements have not been evaluated by the Food and Drug Administration. These products are not intended to diagnose, treat, cure, or prevent a disease.

Below is a list of the most common sexual symptoms and goals, and the nutraceuticals we offer to target them:

Low libido, stamina and/or energy - Beet Vitality, TestroVida Pro, Testrogenesis cream, Power & Speed, Stem Cell Strong, Stay Young AM

Loss of libido in aging adults - Testrogenesis cream, Adrenal DMG, Stem Cell Strong, Stay Young AM, Passion Pill

Loss of libido, arousal or pleasure in conjunction with fatigue and ongoing stress – Adrenal DMG

Reduced arousal and sexual performance caused by narrowed arteries – PCOS Heart Plus, Beet Vitality, Amore V

Erectile dysfunction – PCOS Heart Plus, Beet Vitality

Premature ejaculation (or to delay normal ejaculation) - EstroBlock or DHT Block combined with Liv D-tox and Neuro Insight or Neuro Inspire (to be called Brain Activator)

Male feminization (man boobs etc.) – Estro Block or Estro Block Pro or DHT Block; Liv D-Tox and Neuro Insight

Difficulty achieving orgasm (Female) – Oxytocin, TestroVida Pro, Passion Pill

Lack of lubrication - TestroVida Pro or Testrogenesis cream, Beet Vitality, Stay Young AM

To enhance libido and sexual performance – Beet Vitality, Stem Cell Strong, Amore V, Stay Young AM

For added intensity of pleasure – Passion Pill, Stay Young AM, Amore V

Special occasion sex (for all-night performances, multiple orgasms, and explosive pleasure) – Amore V, Passion Pill

Nutraceuticals for Sexual Health and Virility:

1. TestroVida Pro
2. Testrogenesis Cream
3. Beet Vitality
4. PCOS Heart Plus
5. Estro Block
6. Estro Block Pro
7. Power and Speed
8. Stem Cell Strong
9. Stay Young AM
10. DHT Block
11. Neuro Insight & Neuro Insight (Brain Activator in Doc Nutrients brand)
12. Liv D-Tox

13. Amore V
14. Oxytocin
15. Passion Pill

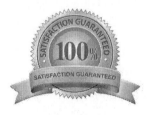

1. TestroVida Pro

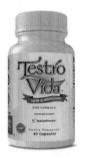

TestroVIda Pro helps to safely and effectively free up bound testosterone, which plays a leading role in sexual desire and pleasure in both males and females. It contains zinc and nearly 20 powerful aphrodisiac herbs (long jack fruit, MACA root, velvet bean, horny goat weed etc.) that not only enhance testosterone production, but also turbocharge libido, and optimize other sex hormone levels. TestroVida Pro also helps support healthy enzymes that prevent the blocking of nitric oxide production. This is helpful for your sex life because nitric oxide plays several key roles in sexual functioning, desire, and arousal.

This product is for you if your testosterone levels are low or on the low end of normal, but you are experiencing sexual symptoms. Common testosterone deficiency symptoms to look out for include a reduced sex drive, loss of libido, delayed or weak orgasms, excess belly fat, muscle loss, inability to lose weight, low mood, and lethargy. Women may also experience vaginal dryness and painful sex, and men may experience reduced sperm volume, weaker erections, and problems with conception.

2. Testrogenesis Cream

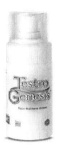

Testrogenesis cream contains 5-A-Hydroxy-Laxogenin which increases the natural production of your free and total testosterone. It also contains the vital hormone for sexual health – DHEA. Declining DHEA levels is one of the reasons why sex often becomes less of a priority in aging adults and restoring youthful levels can dramatically enhance your libido and sex life. DHEA is so important for sexual health because it is a precursor to all of the sex hormones, including testosterone. Using a cream is beneficial because it is absorbed from your skin directly into your bloodstream, bypassing the need for proper digestion and absorption.

Specific herbs have been added to this proprietary formula to improve the release of natural androgens while clearing harmful estrogens and sustaining healthy hormone levels. It also contains DIM to fight estrogen dominance, and zinc to further support healthy testosterone production. This potent cream increases libido in both men and woman, increases energy and stamina, and slows muscle loss and other natural changes in the body that come with age.

3. Beet Vitality

Beet vitality is an exclusive anti-aging formula that can instantly improve your sex life. It contains concentrated beetroot and a proprietary blend of other nutrients that help to

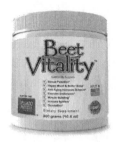

notably boost nitric oxide (NO) levels. This is beneficial because low NO levels cause the blood vessels to restrict which prevents blood flow to the sex organs. Without enough NO, blood flow to the clitoris is inhibited. Increasing NO cannot only enhance sensitivity, but also increase lubrication and make orgasms more intense and easier to achieve for women. Low NO is also a chief cause of erectile dysfunction (ED) in men because NO is required for blood to fill the erectile body, and Beet Vitality can help circumvent this problem.

Many of my patients report increased desire, arousal, and sexual performance on the very first day of starting this exceptional product! As a bonus, it also contains bioavailable protein peptides to help you look and feel years younger; it boosts energy, improves sports performance, stamina, and recovery time; promotes rejuvenating sleep, and helps renew cellular and organ health.

4. PCOS Heart Plus

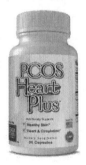

PCOS Heart Plus contains a variety of nutrients that help to lower cholesterol levels, enhance heart health, and reduce arterial plaque build-up. This is important for your sex life because you need a healthy heart and arteries in order for blood to flow to the sex organs. Plaque build-up in the arteries reduces arousal and pleasure sensations and is a major cause of erectile dysfunction. PCOS Heart Plus also helps to stabilize blood sugar and combat metabolic syndrome which is beneficial because there is a strong correlation between diabetes, unstable blood sugar levels and sexual dysfunction.

For this formula, we use a blend of expensive (if you bought them individually), all-natural ingredients to help improve your hormonal, arterial and heart health. You would have to purchase over 6 separate supplements (berberine supplement $36, multivitamin $67, vitamin D supplement $28, probiotic supplement $37, immune system supplement $24, magnesium supplement $24 and even more) at a retail price of over $218 just to equal one bottle of PCOS Heart Plus.

5. Estro Block

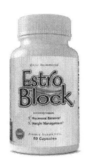

Estro Block is an internationally acclaimed product that helps to balance your hormones and reverse the dangerous and sex sabotaging condition, estrogen dominance. Estrogen dominance is harmful to your sex life because certain forms of estrogen are potent suppressors of testosterone, and the more estrogen you have in your system, the less testosterone you will have available to pump up your sex drive. Estrogen dominance can dull a woman's libido and sabotage her reproductive health. It can take away from a man's masculinity by causing muscle and hair loss, and the development of fatty tissue in the breasts, or "man boobs." It can also cause a reduced ability to achieve erections, lower sperm count, difficult urination, heightened emotional sensitivity, infertility, and premature/rapid ejaculation.

Estro Block is made from natural cruciferous vegetables, it contains clinically effective dosages of DIM and I3C and it is formulated in a way that allows these potent phytochemicals to absorb into the tissues where estrogen dominance resides. Just two capsules of Estro Block per day (one in the morning and one in the evening) offers a concentration of DIM and I3C that is equivalent to eating two pounds of raw cruciferous vegetables. The high doses of absorbable DIM and I3C helps to prevent an enzyme called P450 from converting hormones into more harmful estrogens and androgens.

6. Estro Block Pro

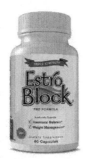

Estro Block Pro contains everything our world renowned Estro Block formula does, plus a whole lot more! This triple strength formula is used by clinicians to fight estrogen dominance and restore hormonal balance. In addition to the extra concentrated doses of DIM and I3C (two extremely potent estrogen reducers), Estro Block Pro also contains chrysin which helps support healthy testosterone levels, and wasabi root and d-glucuronolactone, which help enhance liver function, detoxification and energy.

If you are more than 20 pounds above your ideal weight or suffer with male feminization symptoms you may progress to use Estro Block Pro, starting with one capsule; after one week go to two capsules a day. Women who choose to take Estro Block Pro triple strength, who are no longer cycling, may only require one capsule a day.

7. Power and Speed

A safe, all-natural formula that will dramatically increase energy, alertness, mental clarity, and endurance. Power and

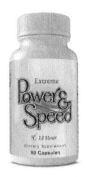

Speed contains a proprietary blend of energy boosting nutrients including guarana, green tea extract, cordyceps, ginseng and kudzu root, which will keep you awake and alert, so you can get through the toughest of workouts or between the sheet sessions. This is a great product if you just don't have the "energy" or drive to engage in sex, and you want a gentle and safe boost.

8. Stem Cell Strong

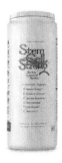

Stem Cell Strong is a potent anti-aging powder that contains nearly 20 powerhouse herbs for optimizing health and restoring a sense of youthful virility. It contains Maca, Long Jack and Velvet Antler to boost testosterone and turbocharge libido; and l-citrulline to enhance blood flow to the sex organs. It also contains a blend of powerful antioxidants to slow the aging process and adaptogenic herbs (ginkgo, ginseng, 5 potent mushrooms etc.) which will boost your energy and stamina both inside and outside of the bedroom.

9. Stay Young AM

This is a great supplement to take daily for enhancing your love life and slowing the aging process. Stay Young AM contains Beetroot, L-Citrulline, Pomegranate, Spinach and Kale powder which help produce a quick and noticeable boost in nitric oxide levels. Many of my clients report a noticeable increase in libido and pleasure sensations immediately after

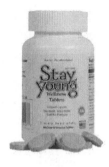

starting this supplement, and women report an increase in lubrication and orgasmic intensity while taking it. It also contains alpha lipoic acid, Coenzyme Q-10, DNA, RNA and phosphatidylcholine to support healthy cells and telomeres, which helps to boost health and vitality.

10. DHT Block

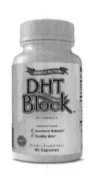

DHT Block contains beta-sitosterol, which gives it the ability to calm down Dihydro-testosterone (DHT) activity in the body and many users report it has helped them to delay ejaculation. DHT Block provides a unique concentration of DIM, isothiocyantates and glucosinolates which help fight estrogen dominance and it's sexual symptoms. It also contains, parsley and celery for cellular and DNA protection, pomegranate to build up the immune system and improve circulation to the sex organs, and astragalus and turmeric to assist with cleansing.

11. Neuro Insight

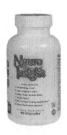

Neuro Insight provides natural and absorbable forms of B12 (methylcobalamin) and 5-methyltetrahydrofolate (folic acid), DMG, MSM, and TMG. These nutrients are important because they provide methyl-donors which are required for methylation. Methylation is important for preventing and reversing estrogen dominance and its sexual symptoms, because it converts estrogens into a form that can be removed from your body, and thereby helps complete the cleansing process.

In addition to fighting estrogen dominance, Neuro Insight also supports healthy brain function, and helps to regulate mood, manage symptoms of PMS, address fibroids, enhance detoxification and combat depression. When combined with DHT Block or Estro Block, it may also help to delay ejaculation.

12. Liv D-Tox

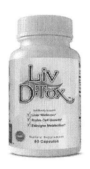

Your liver plays an essential role in over 500 different bodily functions, and your sexual virility and overall wellbeing are intimately connected to the health of your liver. Liver disease is associated with a loss of libido, testicular shrinking, breast enlargement, and a significant reduction of both total and free testosterone levels.

Liv D-Tox is a powerful liver-cleansing supplement. It contains a blend of antioxidant, anti-inflammatory, adaptogenic and liver health promoting herbs including astragalus, turmeric, ginger, oregano, cyprus, asparagus, wasabi and silymarin (milk thistle). When hormones are shifting through their metabolic phases, these herbs tend to move them through their proper pathways, which helps prevent the conversion of testosterone into a variety of harmful estrogens. In so doing, Liv D-Tox helps prevent and reverse estrogen dominance, the negative symptoms associated with testosterone therapy, and with time, it also helps reverse erectile dysfunction caused by estrogen dominance.

13. Amore-V

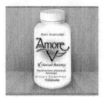 Amore-V is a powerful, safe and all-natural supplement that will allow for mutually mind-blowing sex that lasts all night. It contains a special blend of concentrated herbs that clear enzymes which interfere with nitric oxide (a neurotransmitter that plays a major role in arousal, pleasure and sexual function).

Taken 60 minutes prior to intimacy, this fast-acting pill will turbocharge your sex drive and allow both you and your partner to engage in sex for extended periods of time. It reduces the refractory period between erections and orgasms, enhances vaginal lubrication, and increases clitoral and penile pleasure sensations. Men and women report a fuller romantic experience upon taking the capsule one hour prior to intimate stimulation.

*Amore-V is only available by personal request, and due to its extraordinary popularity, supplies run out fast! To request a bottle, email: Jason@DelgadoProtocol.com or call: 866-319-0566 (toll free in USA) or 1-949-720-1554 (international)

14. Oxytocin

We work with doctors who can prescribe oxytocin. 50 units dissolved under the tongue, 30 minutes prior to sex, can help a woman to more easily reach orgasm and a man to be more loving and relaxed.

15. Passion Pill

Passion Pill is an innovative breakthrough all-natural product for supercharging your sex life. It contains the most powerful blend of nutraceutical ingredients for sexual enhancement available on the market today, including: Herba Epimedii, Rhodiola, Tongkat Ali, Leek Seeds, Tribulus, Wolfberry. A single tablet dissolved under the tongue, taken 90 minutes prior to intimacy, will generate a fuller romantic experience, increase your desire, energy and stamina, enhance blood flow to the sex organs, and bring your pleasure to a higher dimension all night long.

Passion Pill is ideally suited for female physiology of arousal, and it sustains heightened levels of libido and orgasmic intensity, often acting even into the next day. Because Passion PIll takes longer to kick in and tends to remain in action for several hours longer than Amore-V, many men like to take both Amore V and Passion Pill prior to an intimate encounter.

Due to the potency and the proprietary nature of this formula, it is only available by direct email: Rachel@DelgadoProtocol.com or by phone: 866-319-0566 (toll free in USA) or 1-949-720-1554 (international)

Made in the USA
Las Vegas, NV
05 September 2021

29621418R00111